CLASSIC PILATES
METHOD

Centre Yourself with this Step-by-Step Approach
to Joseph Pilates' Original Matwork Programme

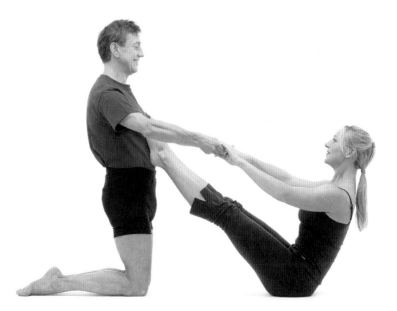

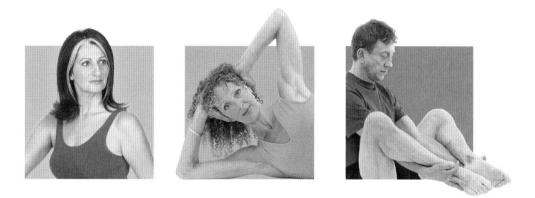

THE COMPLETE

CLASSIC PILATES
METHOD

Centre Yourself with this Step-by-Step Approach
to Joseph Pilates' Original Matwork Programme

by MIRANDA BASS

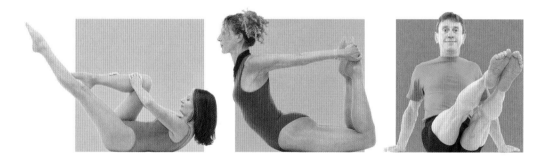

LYNNE ROBINSON   GORDON THOMSON

editor   consultant

MACMILLAN

First published 2004 by Macmillan
an imprint of Pan Macmillan Ltd
Pan Macmillan, 20 New Wharf Road, London N1 9RR
Basingstoke and Oxford
Associated companies throughout the world
www.panmacmillan.com

ISBN 1 4050 0558 0

Text by Miranda Bass

9 8 7 6 5 4 3 2 1

A CIP catalogue record for this book is available from
the British Library.

Typeset by SX Composing DTP, Rayleigh, Essex
Printed and bound in Great Britain by Butler and Tanner

Contents

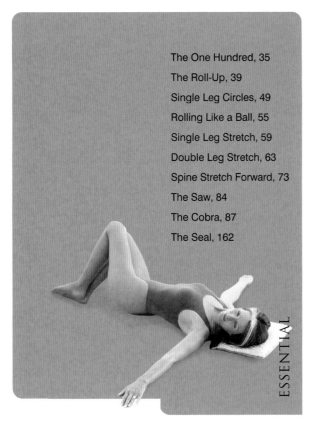

ESSENTIAL

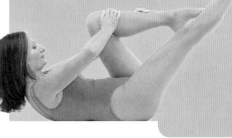

BEGINNERS

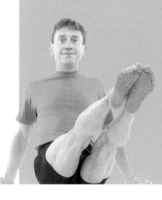

INTERMEDIATE

ADVANCED

About the Author

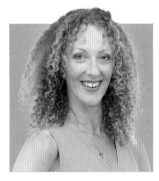

I was first introduced to the Pilates Method by my close friends, Heather and Martin Samson. Heather and I met in 1980 in Mexico when we were on a dancing contract. We kept in touch and, in the early eighties, she opened one of the very first Pilates studios in King's Cross. I was still a professional dancer and visited her studio when I was training in England between contracts. I had suffered an injury to my coccyx right at the beginning of my dancing career which had left me with continual back pain and I found that Pilates not only helped relieve the pain but also kept me in great shape to dance. I wished I had known about it years earlier. These days, most serious dance schools and colleges include Pilates training in their curriculum, mainly as a form of conditioning to prevent the injuries and muscle imbalances so prevalent in dancers and athletes.

I became particularly interested in the mat work because I could practise it on tour in my hotel room, if necessary. At that time, the mat method was little known and studios generally used the machines Joseph Pilates had devised for his conditioning training because, unless mat work is simplified, it is too difficult for the layman.

In 1988, after fourteen years of touring and flogging my body in the dance profession I decided I needed a change and trained in sports injury treatment and massage. At the same time, Heather and Martin trained me as a Pilates teacher in their new studio in Highgate village. I had also qualified in weight training, exercise to music (aerobics), diet and nutrition and anatomy and was working in health clubs and in gyms. I was very loath to leave the world of dance entirely and still did the odd performance here and there. Practising Pilates had greatly improved my dance technique and I was finally pain free. The Pilates Method allowed me to continue dancing in spite of my age! In fact, Pilates was the only form of exercise I really enjoyed and the only one which continued to challenge me. It is similar to classical ballet because it is extremely technical and takes practice. The exercises are choreographed and, as

with dancing, you have to remember the next move.

Slowly, I began to reduce my other work and teach more Pilates classes. My first job as a mat teacher was at Lewisham College. I taught large groups of students on a dance foundation course which was no easy task because they really just wanted to dance and not to exercise. The Pilates Method is not performed to music but to the rhythm of your breath and, unlike dancing, there is little room for self-expression but, once you are well grounded in the technique, and the breath control and placement become automatic, there is room for the sheer enjoyment of movement and control.

I began teaching machine work in various studios in London, including Gordon Thomson's Body Control and Rehabilitation Studio in South Kensington, and for a year I commuted up to the Bedford campus of Middlesex University to train the students on the BA degree course in performing arts. This was one of the most demanding jobs I have ever accepted. I taught Pilates, applied anatomy, dance-injury prevention and coached students with special problems.

This experience taught me a great deal about the uniqueness of the human body and how to adapt the exercises to suit the individual student or client. In those days, the general public knew very little about Pilates mainly because the mat method in its original form was too difficult to teach to groups in a class so we always taught one to one, and not everybody could afford a personal trainer. Today, however, Pilates has become a household name thanks, mainly, to Lynne Robinson and Gordon Thomson who have managed to bring it to a wider audience through their books and videos. To do this, the exercises had to be simplified to a more basic level using elementary movements which allowed the generally unfit a chance to benefit from the mind and body conditioning of the Pilates Method without a private tutor. In consultation with physiotherapists, a type of 'pre-Pilates' has been made available. These basic core exercises are a safe way to introduce some of the principles of the Joseph Pilates Method.

Body Control Pilates Education was set up in 1996 to provide training for people wanting to teach Pilates mat work and machine exercises. The hallmark of the Body Control Pilates approach is the adaptation of the original exercises for the average body, and the development of teachers who instruct on a group basis as opposed to the traditional one-to-one approach. This has been the key element in making the benefits of Pilates accessible to the general public at large as opposed to the elite who lived near a studio and who could afford the cost of private tuition. I joined the team at its inception and have helped to develop several of their courses. I continue to run my own private business in Surrey. My work with Body Control Pilates mainly involves training student teachers at the basic level and then, once they are qualified, helping to advance them to the highest level of the technique and encouraging their further education in subjects such as biomechanics, core stability, anatomy and teaching skills.

Over the years, research into the workings of the human body has made many new discoveries. The sports industry has a vested interest in, and the resources to carry out, continuous research in all aspects of training, injury prevention and, of course, rehabilitation. I find that the research only proves Joseph Pilates to have been way ahead of his time and an expert in body mechanics and rehabilitation. The aesthetics of the Pilates technique, the resulting long, lean muscles and flat firm centre, are an added bonus.

At the close of his book *Your Health* Joseph Pilates says, 'My work will be established and when it is, I will be the happiest man in God's universe. My goal will have been reached.' I have therefore written this book in an attempt to bring the full and original method to light, breaking it down for novices but without losing its essence. In this way, perhaps, I can help to establish Joseph Pilates' work as he taught it, and make him the happiest man in heaven!

There is no doubt it is better to learn with the help of a teacher and, in the past, I have claimed that you cannot learn Pilates from a book. But there are ways to check you are doing the exercises correctly, and I have emphasized this throughout, in detail.

I still practise the method three times a week, alternating mat and reformer work. What I like about the mat method is the fact that you just need your mind, your body and a mat, so there is no excuse for not doing it! You can take it with you anywhere. It takes me approximately 40 minutes to complete the routine without stopping.

Schopenhauer said that 'To neglect one's body for any other advantage in life is the greatest of follies.' Sometimes laziness or fatigue tempt me into not donning my leotard and leggings and getting on with it; after all I have been practising the full mat programme for nearly twenty years. However, I have to practise what I preach (apart from the fact that my back still suffers if I have a break) and once I get going I soon settle into the rhythmical movements and breath control, and always feel revived and rewarded with new energy once I have finished.

Pilates has definitely kept me in good shape, free to move and even to dance again, if I choose. However, one of the greatest things Pilates has given me is self-discipline (vital for someone like me!), a pain-free life and a way to help me focus in this often distracting and confusing world. Many therapies advocate a 'letting go' of oneself in order to find freedom. I believe that freedom, especially to move, comes only through discipline and effort.

My Christian faith, which exercises the spiritual muscles, and Pilates, which exercises the physical muscles and the mind, have helped me overcome depression and injury, among other things, and both have given me an invaluable freedom.

I wish you all the very best in your efforts. Practise faithfully and reap your reward!

God bless you in your endeavours.

'MY AIM IS TO KEEP MOBILE: SO FAR – I AM AGED 86 – PILATES SEEMS TO HAVE PLAYED ITS CONSIDERABLE PART. I MIGHT ADD THAT UNDER THE GUIDANCE OF MIRANDA BASS IT IS NOT ONLY IMMENSELY HELPFUL BUT POSITIVELY ENJOYABLE!'

BETTY JOSEPH, PSYCHOANALYST

To Joseph Pilates, for what he left me,
and which I now pass on to you.

I cannot believe it is nearly two years since I agreed to write this book, when Lynne, Gordon and myself sat in a bar and discussed the approach and the content. It has involved a great deal of hard work and I would like to thank all the team at Pan Macmillan for the colourful and clear presentation of the full mat programme. Many thanks to Lynne and Gordon for introducing me to their publishers and giving me this opportunity.

I could not have written the book without, all my dear clients who have helped me learn how to tailor the exercises to their unique physiques and to find ways of breaking down the exercises when necessary, and for always showing dedication and enthusiasm and a will to learn.

Last but not least I would like to acknowledge my own teachers: Heather and Martin Samson, who introduced me to Pilates; Siri Dharma, a teacher who gives her all, who has a great knowledge and who continues to challenge me and make it fun. To Michael Miller who gave me a new inspiration and hosted a wonderful Pilates tour from Denver to Seattle, which was unforgettable.

Miranda Bass

I would like to express my deepest gratitude to, and admiration for, the network of Body Control Pilates teachers and support staff who continue to overwhelm us with their enthusiasm, professionalism and thirst for knowledge. Each and every one has helped us realize the vision we had when we created the Body Control Pilates Method some eight years ago. I look forward to an exciting future as we continue to find new ways to challenge and develop our teachers still further!

I would also especially like to thank Miranda for agreeing to write the book and for helping to create a programme that is a natural progression from the earlier Body Control Pilates books. This is destined to become a standard reference manual in the Pilates world.

Lynne Robinson

I would like to dedicate my part in this book to the memory of my mother who passed away suddenly and tragically during editing. I was looking forward to giving her one of the first copies because she has always been an inspiration and encouragement to me – I hope Dad can gain some comfort from seeing the project come to fruition.

My thanks go to Miranda and Lynne with whom I have enjoyed working on this book, and to the editorial team at Macmillan (Gordon Wise and Rafi Romaya) who have moulded our contributions into such an elegant product. Above all, cheers and thanks to the whole Body Control Pilates tradition. This book – like all the others which have gone before – has been made possible by the magic which colleagues bring to our endeavour. The Association offers us a worldwide network of brilliant and challenging disciples. My own studio in South Kensington gives me personal support and a sense of purpose which I cannot imagine doing without – thank you to my clients, friends and especially to Cheryl, Ellie, Judy, Patricia, Fran, Lawrence and Richard. Last but not least – as the expression goes – Body Control has produced a succession of beautiful, super-fit models whom the reader of this and previous manuals should enjoy following in their every move!

Gordon Thomson

The Man, The Method, The Moment

The Man with a Vision

Joseph Pilates, the creator of this proven method is, sadly, no longer with us. He died in 1967 at the age of eighty-seven from smoke inhalation, the result of a fire in his New York studio. He was in fantastic physical shape at the time of his death and could perform his method with grace and ease.

Little is known of his background or his family except that he was born in 1880 into a working-class family in Düsseldorf, Germany. He is reported to have suffered from several childhood diseases associated with poverty: rheumatic fever, asthma and rickets. These illnesses would have left Joseph Pilates weak, underdeveloped and with a fear of developing the structural deformities associated with these ailments in the long term.

A form of physical training had just been introduced into schools in Germany, so perhaps his initiation into physical fitness began there. His mother, allegedly, practised some sort of alternative medicine and perhaps this also influenced him. He must have had tremendous willpower and determination to overcome his early frailty because, by the age of fourteen, he had managed to re-build his body enough to be able to pose for anatomical drawings.

During the 1890s and the early 1900s a new awareness of health through exercise was springing up. Discoveries about the workings of the body and the mind were leading various doctors, scientists and writers to explore weight training, gymnastics and all other forms of physical conditioning and their effects on the health of both the mind and the body.

Through the transformation of his own body and the influences of these new ideas, Joseph Pilates devised his method and adopted a philosophy based on that of the ancient Greeks, embodied by the Latin saying, *mens sana in corpore sano* (a sound mind in a healthy body).

Joseph came to England in about 1912 and worked as a boxer and circus performer. He became involved with teaching detectives in the English police force but when war broke out he was interned in Lancaster and later, on the Isle of Man. He is reputed to have become a nurse and went on developing his method with other internees. At the time there was a particularly nasty influenza epidemic and his method was praised when none of the internees became infected. While he was still interned he designed the reformer by using the bed springs as an exercise unit, utilizing the tension of the springs to strengthen wasted muscle.

After the war he moved to New York and set up a studio which he ran with his wife, Clara, a former nurse. Their success in restoring weak and sickly bodies was soon renowned. His technique particularly attracted people in the worlds of the performing arts and medicine. He took on apprentices and it is through them that his method has spread internationally, gradually at first and now with huge momentum!

Pilates definitely meant his method to be available to everyone and he published his own book, *Return to Life Through Contrology*. (Joseph Pilates referred to his method as Contrology, nowadays we call it the Pilates Method.) He could see that modern living, particularly in a city, was having a disastrous effect on people's health and fitness levels. He thought there was a clear connection between poor posture, sedentary life-styles and ill health. He studied many types of body conditioning, including bodybuilding and yoga – the latter was just sweeping into the West – and he found weight training and the usual forms of strengthening and stretching boring and monotonous, and realized they had the potential to make you stiff and tired. The Pilates Method uses very few repetitions but encourages a flow of motion by a continuous changing of positions. You have to engage your entire body and focus your mind during each exercise in order to coordinate the movements. Pilates said, 'One of the major results of Contrology is gaining the mastery of your mind over the complete control of your body.'

Since its inception the Pilates Method has been referred to as a form of mental and physical conditioning and is a great deal more than just a workout. Pilates claimed that 'Contrology develops the body uniformly, corrects wrong postures, restores physical vitality, invigorates the mind and elevates the spirit.'

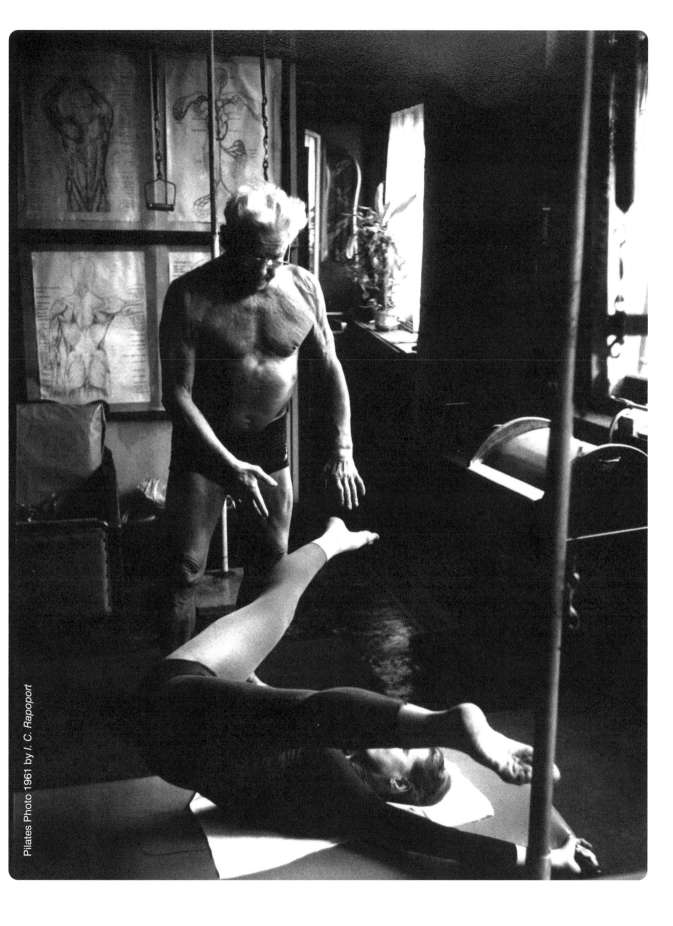

The Method

The Pilates Method is a type of physical and mental conditioning using well-designed, choreographed movements properly performed and in a balanced sequence. The emphasis is not on quantity but on quality. It is a mindful form of exercise where each movement is performed consciously, with slow control and with a particular breathing pattern. The complete mat method works every muscle group in the body with special attention to the muscles which stabilize the joints, thus producing correct body mechanics, economy of energy expenditure and a uniform flow of energy channelled through the entire body. Joseph Pilates designed specialized machines, using the tension of springs, and these exercises are generally referred to as the 'studio work'. Some of the machine work was designed to help people towards achieving the exercises performed on the mat. In this book I have broken down some of the repertoire to help you slowly build up the strength you need to perform the full programme.

'TO THE UNEDUCATED EYE, PILATES MOVEMENTS MAY LOOK SIMPLE. NOT ONLY DO THEY OFFER PHYSICAL BENEFITS; THE CONCENTRATION REQUIRED TONES THE CONSCIOUSNESS AS WELL. FOR ME, STUDYING PILATES HAS CONTRIBUTED TO CREATING A UNION BETWEEN THE BODY AND MIND. THIS IN TURN HAS INCREASED MY CAPACITY FOR CONCENTRATION. AS A RESULT, I FEEL MORE CENTRED, IN BODY, MIND AND SPIRIT. AND IT TEACHES BALANCE, THE KIND THAT'S VITAL FOR DESK-BOUND WRITERS – AND IS A REAL BONUS WHEN MANOEUVRING IN SPINDLY HIGH HEELS . . .'

SHELLY VON STRUNCKEL, ASTROLOGER.

The Mind

Each exercise at every level requires a huge amount of concentration. Your mind controls your body and the programme makes you aware of this ultimate control and demands you use it. It will never be easy, but eventually the correct breathing, abdominal control, shoulder stabilization and coordination which are all essential to performing the exercises correctly should become second nature. It's like learning to drive a car or a bicycle – you always have to concentrate and make an effort but some aspects become automatic.

Pilates' desire was that we become more aware of our subconscious behavioural patterns, not just our physical or muscular behaviour, but mental and emotional as well. He explained that, 'First you purposefully acquire complete control of your body and then, through proper repetition of Contrology exercises you gradually and progressively acquire that natural rhythm and coordination associated with all your subconscious activities.'

You will not be able to do the programme very well to start with but, through effort and discipline you will reap the reward. It is, and should continue to be, a challenge. You have aims to strive for and it is with the accomplishment of these aims that you will gain the self-confidence and empowerment that Pilates talked of: 'Self-confidence, poise [and] consciousness of possessing the power to accomplish our desires with renewed vigor and interest in life.'

His interpretation of physical fitness begins with the mind: 'The attainment and maintenance of a uniformly developed body with a sound mind, fully capable of naturally, easily and satisfactorily performing our many daily tasks with spontaneous zest and pleasure.' Joseph Pilates was aware that over time the repetition of his movements formed new nerve pathways in the brain, awakening and stimulating the mind.

What the method teaches you to do is to focus. In this age of technology with everything speeding up to a frenetic level, focusing is hard. Practising Pilates helps you settle your mind, enabling you to achieve your purpose, and this skill can be applied to any area of life, work, relationships, sport and recreation.

The Body

The spine takes precedence in the Pilates Method. 'Rolling up and rolling down through the spine with correct breathing requires persistence and earnest effort but it is worth it.'

Joseph Pilates knew that a stiff spine makes you feel old. Even if your limbs are fine, if you can't move or control your spine – the centre core of the body – effectively, the limbs will not function as they should. Segmental control of the spine is one of the first requirements of the Pilates Mat Method.

Pilates spoke of 'the powerhouse', the large powerful group of muscles at the very centre of the body which move and stabilize the trunk and pelvis. All movement emanates from them. If there is control and stability at the centre, movement flows out from it easily. You learn to channel your energy and synchronize your muscle activity with the minimum amount of effort, leaving the limbs and extremities free of tension. You will acquire physical grace.

His special emphasis on correct and conscious breathing is an integral part of the method and aids the movements. The breathing is demanding and, ultimately, aerobic once you have learnt the exercises and can do them without stopping which makes the blood pump through the body. Pilates wanted to wash the blood completely with clean oxygen so it reached every part of the body. He called this 'an internal shower'.

He was very conscious of the connections between the structure of the body and its internal organs and one of the reasons the method is performed lying down, for the most part, is to remove stress from the heart, allow the organs to settle and reprogramme the postural muscles without the normal pull of gravity.

Pilates had a holistic approach to health and was a forerunner in physical education. He envisioned that everyone would learn to be conscious of how their body worked and would train it to combat the effects of modern living, and return to the natural rhythms of movement we have strayed from in our industrial, and now technological, age.

The essence of the Pilates technique is simultaneously to strengthen and lengthen the body and have complete control over it. You stretch the spine using the abdominals and, conversely, stretch the abdominals using the muscles of the back; the hamstrings are stretched using the powerful hip flexors; the hip flexors by using the buttocks and hamstrings and so on. This is called 'dynamic stretching' and is proving to be a safe and functional way to increase flexibility. What is the point of having long, stretched hamstrings at the back of the leg, if the opposite muscles, the quadriceps and hip flexors, cannot take the leg to that range of motion?

During the programme you will use every muscle in the body as you reorganize your posture. Because so many exercises are performed lying down, reprogramming postural abnormalities and bad habits is easier. In many exercises, gravity is used as a weight and you use your muscles to combat its pull. Working the muscles while you lengthen them is also an integral part of the training. We call this an 'eccentric contraction' of a muscle or muscle group, and recent research shows this to be more powerful than a concentric contraction, when the muscle shortens as it contracts.

Generally, the physical workout you get from Pilates is challenging, uniform, strengthening and mobilizing, and very modern in spite of its age!

The Spirit

Joseph Pilates called the spirit 'the gheist', the ghost or spirit. He thought that a type of spiritual peace could be obtained by practising his method. He didn't claim it gives salvation, although he spoke of his Creator and obviously believed in God. However, the discipline, the joy of movement and the awareness of the miracle of the human body can all help lift our spirits.

There is no doubt that exercise changes our biochemistry and produces chemicals that give a sense of well-being and even euphoria. Perhaps this is the 'gheist' that Joseph Pilates refers to. Your spirits will be raised by the method because you have the discipline to treat your body to a healthy conditioning and to overcome initial failure.

'THE IDEAL TO STRIVE FOR IS THE
ENJOYMENT OF PHYSICAL WELL-BEING,
MENTAL CALM AND SPIRITUAL PEACE.
IN OUR OPINION IT IS ONLY THROUGH
CONTROLOGY THAT THIS UNIQUE TRINITY
OF A BALANCED BODY, MIND AND SPIRIT
CAN EVER BE OBTAINED.'

JOSEPH PILATES

The Principles of the Technique

Concentration
This is the first requirement and none of the other principles can be achieved without this focusing of the mind over the body. Once you have learnt the movements there is a danger you will slip into poor technique. Keep reading through the check points at the end of each exercise. They explain what you need to concentrate on by pointing out common faulty movements and the ways in which the body likes to cheat!

Control
Each movement is controlled and never thrown away. If you start to lose control, stop and go on to the next exercise. As you practise you will gain the strength and mental ability to control the number of repetitions specified. The movements should be performed within a controlled range within which you can keep your alignment and stability.

Centring
This is the ability to find and use the powerhouse, discussed earlier on page 5. Every single exercise requires this ability. Our centre of gravity lies very low, just below the point where the pelvis meets the spine. The muscles stabilizing this area are transversus abdominus, a deep abdominal muscle which draws the abdomen in towards the spine but does not move the bones, and multifidus, deep spinal muscles which run up the length of the spine, fine-tuning the movements of the trunk. The muscles controlling the powerhouse are the big hip flexors, the buttocks, the superficial abdominals and the muscles in the lower back. From this central area movement emanates and correct centring and use of these muscles should lead to the next principle – flowing movement.

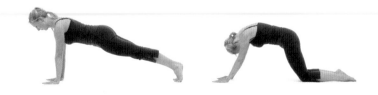

Flowing Movement

For a movement to flow, all the muscles required for that movement need to work together. Apart from the main movers there are many other muscles involved in the actions we make. For example, when picking up a shopping bag from the floor, the biceps (the agonist) contract as you bend the arm to lift the bag. On the back of the arm the triceps (antagonists) are having to lengthen to allow the arm to bend and help control the pace of the movement. The muscles in the shoulder work to keep the shoulder from being displaced by the weight, as do the muscles in the wrist. These are acting as joint stabilizers. There are also other muscles working in the arm to keep the movement in one plane. These are the neutralizers or synergists. When learning a new movement these muscles have to learn when to start contracting so the action is performed smoothly. At first you might find you are a little jerky and uncoordinated but after practising for a while, your brain will become accustomed to the order of the instructions it needs to send to the appropriate muscles and you will acquire the desired flow. However, if your alignment is incorrect, your centre weak or your muscles unfit, it will affect your ability to achieve this flowing movement with grace.

Breathing

Breath control is an integral part of the technique. It is the first thing your mind has to focus on. This helps you internalize, to get inside your body and begin to control muscles you have probably never even considered, muscles which are controlled subconsciously. It puts you in touch with yourself and initiates the idea of regaining control of automatic and habitual behaviour.

However, that is not all. The emphasis Joseph Pilates placed on how to breathe is vital to actually getting through the exercises. The programme requires a good deal of effort even though you only do a few repetitions of each exercise and you are moving fairly slowly. If you do not breathe properly you will tire, and your muscles will ache.

The breathing patterns aid the movements. For example, curling up through the spine from lying, trunk flexion, is facilitated by exhalation, while bending the spine backwards, trunk extension, is facilitated by inhalation. Learn the breathing patterns, remembering that the inhalation is in the back of the ribcage and not in the lower abdominals. Always exhale completely; emptying the lungs aids in cleansing your system. The deep stabilizer of the pelvis, transversus abdominus, which plays a role in maintaining intra-abdominal pressure, aids in forcing exhalation. Emptying the lungs is important to the technique.

Precision

The exercises are described in detail in the book with pictures as visual aids and, if possible, your own image in a mirror to help you. Be conscious of every part of your body and check yourself continually from head to toe. Know where your body is going. Be definite and accurate in your movements, working on correct placement and coordination without losing fluidity and grace.

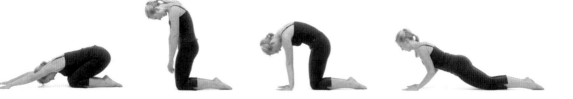

The Moment

So where is the Pilates Method today? This book represents a close portrayal of the original Pilates Mat Method. There are many books and videos on the market claiming to represent Pilates' exercises, but much of this material is not the Pilates Method as Joseph Pilates taught it but adaptations based on various other therapeutic exercises. There is nothing wrong with the exercises portrayed in these books, but they rarely present the original method. The order, number of repetitions and technique of the full mat programme are essential ingredients to the exercises actually achieving what they are supposed to.

The Body Control Pilates organization has already published several books on the Pilates Method, including *Body Control the Pilates Way*, *Pilates the Way Forward* and *The Official Body Control Pilates Manual*. The emphasis of these books has been mainly on rehabilitation and therapeutic exercise. They explain the basic principles of the method, for example body awareness, basic core stability, shoulder stabilization and breath control. The exercises are broken down into elementary movements so as to lead people carefully into the method without causing injury. As you will discover, the programme in its completeness, as described in this book, is hard to achieve and results in a high level of fitness. This book is suitable for people who are virtually pain free and over twelve years old up to any age. I hope the instructions will also be useful to teachers of the method.

You can continue with any other sports or exercise while doing Pilates because it will improve your performance in all forms of movement as a result of its emphasis on correct body mechanics and balance between strength and flexibility with conscious control.

As a result of recent studies, the method has been refined and slightly modified to fall in line with new discoveries about body mechanics. However, for the most part, the research only proves that Joseph Pilates was way ahead of his time and had an extraordinary insight into biomechanics.

The science is therefore well established, but Pilates described his method, time and time again as 'an art and a science'. There is much more to it than just using the body correctly. The grace of flowing movement, the control and the centring of mind and body require the practice and skill required of say, a dancer, a painter or a singer. It is partly this conscious and creative discipline that makes the Pilates Method unique and has continued to acquire it disciples for nearly a century and which continues to increase its popularity daily.

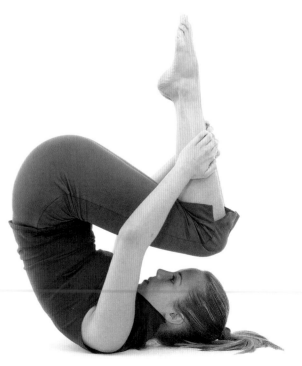

'HAVING EXERCISED AT A
GYM FOR MANY YEARS, I WAS
RECENTLY INTRODUCED TO
PILATES. I FOUND THAT
AFTER ONLY A FEW LESSONS,
MY BODY HAS BECOME MORE
SUPPLE, MY STOMACH IS
FLATTER AND I FEEL MORE
FLUID AND LITHE. I FEEL
THAT I'VE DISCOVERED A
METHOD OF EXERCISE THAT
ALLOWS ME TO RELAX AND
ACHIEVE IMPRESSIVE RESULTS
AT THE SAME TIME.
I NOW RECOMMEND PILATES
TO ALL MY CLIENTS, BECAUSE
I FEEL THAT THEY WILL NOT
ONLY ENJOY THE CLASSES,
BUT ALSO SEE REAL RESULTS.
I WISH I HAD STARTED
YEARS AGO!'

IAN MARBER, NUTRITIONIST

How To Use This Book

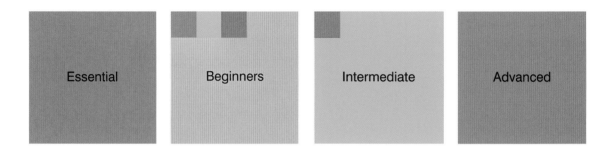

Essential   Beginners   Intermediate   Advanced

The levels have been coded, for ease of reference, using a coloured border; yellow for beginners; green for intermediate; red for advanced. If an exercise is for more than one level an appropriately coloured box has been included in the border.

It is very difficult to teach yourself Pilates, but I have done my best to give the reader as many aids as possible. Although you can see the positions from the pictures it is hard to know if you are copying them properly. This is why I have suggested using a mirror or another pair of eyes. We might think we are positioned correctly but we are often far too familiar and comfortable in our poor postures and faulty movement patterns to be sure. Strictly speaking, Pilates cannot be properly learnt from a book but if you are going to try, this is the book to use. The exercises have been broken down into three levels – beginners, intermediate and advanced – but without changing the essence of each exercise. In this way, the integrity of the method has been maintained and will lead you carefully through each level to the full programme.

Everyone must start with the Fundamentals of the Pilates Technique on page 15. This section teaches you how to be aware of correct alignment and joint stabilization. Once you have learned this essential awareness of your own body you must learn the Warm-Up on page 23. You will not understand the language used in the instructions for the programme if you try to miss out any of these preparatory exercises. The Warm-Up should *always* be done before you start on the actual programme, no matter what level you have achieved, because it gently lengthens the spine and gets the mind connected to the body, and particularly to the transversus abdominus, to prepare you for the more demanding exercises.

Whatever level of fitness you possess, you *must* start with the beginners' versions of the exercises. You should do the few essential beginners' exercises first, these are indicated by a blue box on the yellow beginners' border, then add one or two more beginners' exercises at a time in the order they are in the book. It will be a 'stop and start' process at first because you will have to refer continuously to the book and this is time-consuming – persevere! Once you are familiar with each movement, try and work without the book so you can flow from one exercise to the next. The essential exercises should not take more then 10 to 15 minutes once you know them.

When you can perform the beginners' programme correctly and with increasing ease, move on to the intermediate programme. It is difficult to gauge how long this process takes, but through experience of teaching I estimate six months to a year depending on your body type, mental control, flexibility and strength (less for dancers and gymnasts). You might have to remain with the beginners' versions of some of the exercises for some time while moving on to a higher level for others. People's bodies are different: you might be great at rolling up through the spine but find the back or leg extensions difficult.

The beginners' programme does not include set transitions. These are only included for the intermediate and advanced versions. These transitions explain how to get from one posture to the next, adding a flow to the routine of the exercises and helping you keep the mind focused and the body alert. Leaving a gap and constant pauses between the exercises reduces the stamina we are aiming to achieve and breaks the concentration level.

Try the intermediate versions of all the exercises and then practise them until you are absolutely sure of what you are doing and you find the exercises are becoming easy. Then you can start on the advanced programme. It may take a long time to achieve this level but this is your challenge. Because flexibility plays a large role in the full mat method and some people may never achieve it, you can stick to some of the intermediate versions while moving on to the advanced versions for other exercises. Whatever version you are doing you go on practising it with dedication and precision and in good faith, perfecting it more each time.

Once you have learnt the movements and can practise without constantly referring to the book, keep the book by your side so you can revise the check points and examine yourself for faulty or bad habits.

I have not described the anatomy of the body or included pictures of the exact muscles being emphasized because I want students to comprehend the 'feel' of the movement. You need to be aware of every part of your body throughout each exercise and not isolate one muscle group. Use the photographs, your eyes on your own body and its reflection in a mirror to help you understand how to do the exercises. Keep going over the check points; check yourself from head to toe all the time.

Main Pointers

- You should read the book through first without doing any of the exercises. This will give you a mental picture of what you are going to do and the exercises will start to sink into your mind and that part of your brain which learns movement patterns. You will notice that many check points are repeated over and over again throughout the programme. These must be embedded in your mind.

- It is essential you follow the instructions exactly as they are laid out.

- Look carefully at each picture; they act as visual instructions. Try and copy the shape made by the body and pay attention to details, such as the positioning of the head, hands and feet.

- Use the mirror to check your posture but only for a moment. Adjust whatever you see is out of place or asymmetrical, then look straight ahead and 'feel' the position or movement. You must know what it feels like when it is right. Throughout the programme you are checking for body symmetry and correct alignment! Unfortunately, for technical reasons, we were unable to use a mirror in the majority of the photographs.

- You could embark on this challenge with a friend or partner. You really need a second pair of eyes. You check each other through each exercise using the check points.

Items You Will Need

- A medium-sized, lightweight mirror (two if possible – one face on and the other in profile) which you can move round. The mirror is essential for checking alignment. We are very rarely in the position we think we are in and more often than not are one-sided. You should always look for body symmetry. Where appropriate, the position of the mirror/mirrors is indicated in the exercises. Study yourself carefully.
- A good quality exercise mat. Ultimately you will need a wide mat so you can roll over without coming off it. You need a high-density foam one especially if you are working on a wooden floor and not a carpet.
- A flat cushion for head support or a small folded towel. Not everyone needs one.
- A large space in which you can move freely, which is fairly warm and removed from any disturbances – telephone, television, family or exterior noises. You must not feel cramped, because you have to extend out of your joints and your centre. Your concentration is very important, so put the answering machine on and tell your partner and children you are not to be disturbed unless it is an emergency!
- Time in the week to practise for three or four sessions. Mark your diary with the times you will practise. At first you should do four short sessions. Remember, this is about self-discipline!
- Once proficient, you should do two or three longer sessions a week. Be strict with yourself!

What You Need to Wear

- You must be able to see your body. Awareness of your body, of your posture and of how you are moving is essential to gaining the full benefits of the programme. Women should wear a leotard or body and leggings or tights. A well-fitted T-shirt will suffice, but it must fit to your skin and allow freedom of movement. Men have less choice. Cycling shorts are the ideal leg wear. Ordinary shorts can prohibit some of the movements and are rarely fitted well enough. A pair of tracksuit bottoms and a T-shirt, which fit well, are suitable. It is best to have bare feet or wear socks. If your feet slide in some of the advanced exercises, take your socks off.
- You should tie your hair up in order to see your head and neck alignment. However, make sure the pony tail or bun is not prohibiting the placement of the back of the skull on the mat or head support.
- Remove your jewellery. Rings may hurt when clasping the hands together, necklaces and earrings can get in the way and be dangerous.

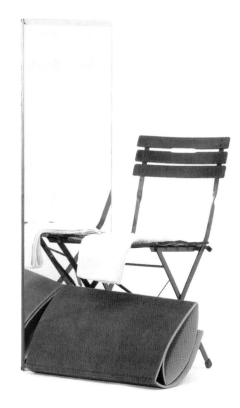

Warning

→ If you have any doubts about practising the Pilates Method please consult your medical practitioner. The exercises have been set out in such a way as to make them safe. The idea is to build up strength and flexibility slowly. Follow the instructions carefully and do not try and run before you can walk! As described in the text on the method, the technique has many benefits for general health issues but you must listen to your body. If it hurts it is a sign that either your technique is incorrect or the exercise is unsuitable for you. If any of the exercises cause you pain then omit them. However, do not confuse pain with effort!

The Fundamentals of the Pilates Technique

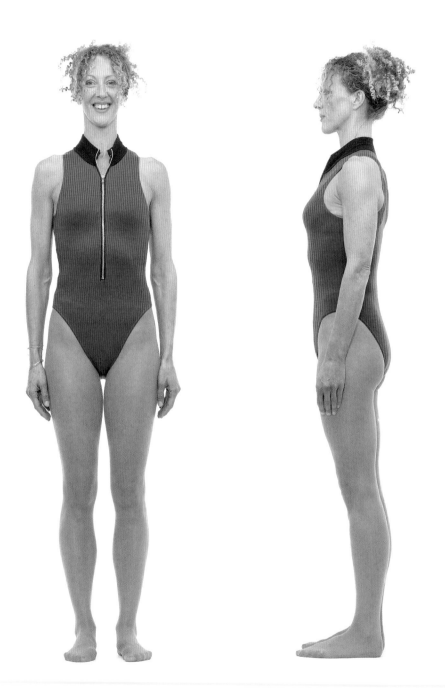

Head, Neck, Shoulder, Pelvic, Leg, Knee and Foot Alignment

It is no use exercising if you are not using correct body mechanics. Yes, you will burn energy, you will tone muscle and you will exercise your heart and lungs, but if your alignment is not right, your biomechanics won't be right either, and you are likely to end up doing more harm than good, whatever form of exercise you have chosen. Correct alignment is one of the most challenging and important parts of any exercise programme.

Whether you are standing, sitting, lying down on your back or on your side, the same alignment applies and the position of your body should be as if a plumbline were running through the centre of it.

To check your alignment when standing use a full-length mirror to look at your head, spine, pelvic and leg alignment from the side. You will have to turn your head, so it is difficult to judge if the tip of your ear is in line with the centre of your shoulder, as it should be, but you should be able to detect if you have the forward head line so common today due to working at a desk and in front of a VDU. The chin should be parallel to the floor and there should be a feeling of length through the back of the neck. From the centre of your shoulder, the plumbline should divide the ribcage in half and then pass just behind the hip joint and on through the knee behind the kneecap, dropping down to just in front of the outside of the ankle bone.

The pelvis should not be dropped forward, giving a pronounced arch to the back, neither should it be tucked under, flattening the lumbar arch. You can check the position of the pelvis by placing the hands in a diamond shape across it and making sure that the pubic bone and the two hip bones are in the same vertical plane. Our bodies are designed to carry the head directly over the shoulders and the shoulders over the pelvis and our centre of gravity.

Take a good look at your posture straight on and notice any asymmetry.

- Is your head to one side or slightly rotated?
- Are your shoulders level?
- How do your arms hang?
- Are your hips level?
- Are you standing with your weight evenly distributed between both feet?
- Leg Alignment. Are your toes pointing forward or do they turn outwards on one or both legs? There should be a straight line running up from your second toe, through the centre of your kneecap and on up to a point 5 or 6 centimetres in from the hip bone. Keeping the knee in line with the second toe is important during all activity. The knee joint is captured between our body weight and the ground and poor lower leg alignment can lead to knee problems and pain which can transfer into the hips and ultimately the spine. Remember to align the legs while doing the exercises. The same alignment applies even if the legs are turned out.Try and find a symmetry, and then feel what you are doing to maintain it. Do not force anything. Use a minimal amount of effort to find a balanced and comfortable position. It may feel strange because you are not used to it, but, if practised enough, it will soon feel right.

Lateral or Thoracic Breathing

It is very important to protect the spine during the exercises and this means you must learn how to breathe into the ribcage and not into the lower abdominals. which are activated to help protect and support the lower back. This breathing technique is often one of the most difficult parts of the Pilates Method to achieve because breathing is a subconscious activity.

Weak abdominals will lead to decreased lung capacity. The ribcage surrounds the lungs and should open and close with each breath. Some people breathe into the upper chest and others into the lower abdominals. See which type of 'breather' you are and keep practising this lateral breathing technique and apply it during each exercise.

The easiest way to practise is from a four-point-kneeling position.

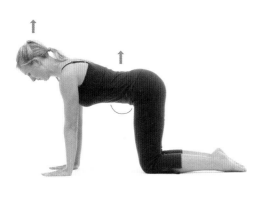

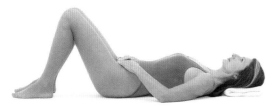

Aim

To practise breathing into the back of the ribcage while supporting the spine in neutral with transversus abdominus.

Starting Position

Assume a four-point-kneeling position on the mat. Place the hands under the shoulders and the knees under the hips. Look down straight between your hands and press the back of the skull up towards the ceiling. Lengthen the tailbone away so your spine is in the neutral position, see page 21. The pelvis should be parallel with the floor; the pubic and two hip bones level with the floor.

Movement

- Breathe in and let the lower abdominals fill with air so they lower towards the floor.
- Breathe out and, as you slowly control the exhalation, draw the lower abdominals in towards the spine. The trunk and pelvis should not move. Check your profile in the mirror. You should just see the stomach pulling up to the spine.
- Repeat this 3 or 4 times. Then try breathing in and out, opening and closing the ribs, without letting the lower abdominals drop down. Keep the navel in to the spine. You might not be able to breathe in very deeply at first.
- Do up to 10 breaths and rest.

You should then practise sitting or kneeling up with your hands around the lower ribs, feeling for the ribcage movement. Finally, practise in the Relaxation Position (page 21) where you spread the ribs sideways across the mat, like breaking open a waistcoat.

Check Points

- Use the mirror or put one hand on the lower abdominals to check for unwanted movement.
- The head, neck and chest should remain calm.
- The spine and pelvis do not move.

Shoulder Stabilization

There are instructions throughout the programme to 'keep the gap between the collarbone and the ear' and 'to fix the shoulders down the back'. The two main shoulder stabilizing muscles keep the shoulder blades down the back and hold them lying snugly against the ribs. When weight-bearing on the hands these muscles have to work hard, for example during Push-Up, or the Twist (pages 172 and 155).

At other times they have to work with less intensity, for example, during the Double Leg Stretch (page 63), when the arms circle up and round. During any exercise involving a sit-up or a curl-up the shoulders are likely to curl forwards and rise up towards the ears. You need to keep an eye on yourself and guard against hunching the shoulders during any of the exercises.

The following exercise is a way to find and strengthen the shoulder stabilizers.

Chair Dips

Aim
To strengthen the shoulder stabilizers.

Starting Position
Sit up straight on the edge of the seat of a sturdy dining-room chair. Hold on to the front edge of the seat with your hands. Bend the elbows if necessary to draw the collarbones away from the ears. The mirror should be face on to you.

Movement
- Breathe out and walk the feet slightly out in front of you so you are just off the seat. Keep the collarbones away from the ears as you take your weight on your hands and feet. Keep your hips on the same level as the seat.
- Breathe in and hold the position keeping the shoulders down.
- Breathe out and walk back to sit down again, maintaining shoulder stabilization.
- Do up to 10 repetitions.

Check Points
- Do not walk out too far, only enough to get the buttocks off the chair.
- If your wrists hurt, try holding the front corners of the seat so you can turn the wrists outwards a little.
- Keep pushing down into the seat with the hands lifting up through the crown of the head.
- Keep your head in line with your shoulders.

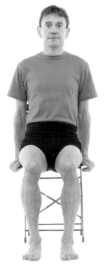
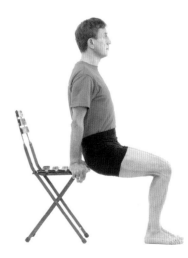

Pelvic and Lumbar Stabilization

Our spines form in one long curve as we lie curled snugly in the womb. After birth, as we develop the strength to function against the force of gravity, we acquire two inward curves, one in the neck, as we learn to support our heads, and the other in the lower back, as we learn to sit up and walk. These curves are important for shock absorption and balance. Sometimes these curves can become distorted through poor postural examples learnt from our parents, through sedentary life styles or because of injury or sickness. There are many common distortions: flat backs, where the curves disappear; lordosis, where the lumbar curve becomes exaggerated: scoliosis, where there is a sideways curve like a 'C' or a double curve like an 'S'.

Our aim is to maintain the gentle curves of a natural or neutral spine. Because the weight of the body presses downwards, the lumbar curve is often the most vulnerable and most likely to suffer change. The junction where the spine meets the pelvis, the lumbar-sacral joint where the fifth and last lumbar vertebra meets the sacrum, is particularly at risk, so we must also look at the neutral or natural position of the pelvis.

Getting Straight on Your Mat

It is very important that you lie in the centre of your mat so you can use it like a grid to check your alignment and to help guide both sides of the body, to work equally. Some of the rolling exercises particularly will reveal an imbalance, weakness or tightness in one side. Use the mat as a frame for your body.

- Sit towards the end of the mat and bend the knees up, placing your feet on the floor hip-width apart. Use the edge of the mat as a guide. With your hands on the mat shift your sit bones towards your heels so they are lined up. Your sit bones are the two bony projections of the pelvis you can feel under the fleshy part of your bottom. (If you are sitting up correctly on a chair with a firm seat you will feel where these bones are. If you are slumped when seated you will roll back on to the end of the spine instead of finding that balance on the bottom of the pelvis.)
- Place your hands behind you and use them to help you roll down slowly through the spine. Then settle into the Relaxation Position.

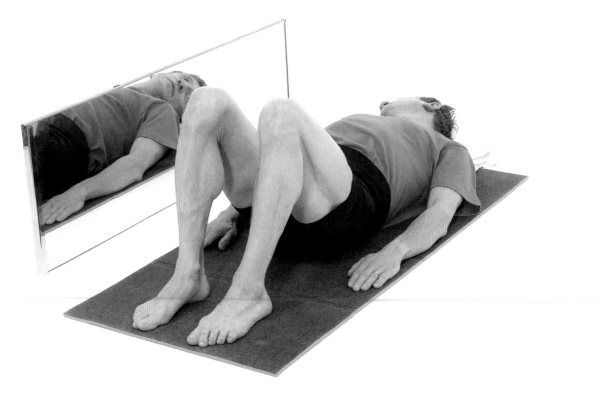

Relaxation Position: Finding Neutral Spine and Pelvis

- When lying in the Relaxation Position, the first position to be learnt, the back of the skull should be resting on the mat and the chin should be parallel to the floor. If your head tips back and you cannot maintain the correct positioning, use a small folded towel or a flat cushion under the head.
- The thoracic spine, where the ribs join the vertebrae which run from the top of the shoulders through to just above the waistline, should be supported on the mat.
- The lumbar spine should be off the mat, so you can slide the hands flat through the small gap on the floor under your waist to the back of the hip crests. Most people will let the lower back drop into the floor but you must practise maintaining these gentle, natural curves in the back.
- The pelvis should be balanced on the end of the spine. We refer to this as the tailbone, although the actual tailbone, or coccyx, curves inwards towards the anus and it is really the end of the sacrum you feel on the mat. You can check the position of the pelvis by making sure the pubic bone and the two hip bones are on the same transverse plane. If you put a small plate on your lower abdomen, across the pelvic area, and then placed a marble on the plate, the marble would not roll anywhere.
- In the Relaxation Position, the heels are in line with the sit bones and the feet point straight forward. The knees point straight up to the ceiling and the thigh bones drop down into the hip sockets in parallel lines.

Note

The hip sockets are set in from the hip bones by approximately 4 to 6 centimetres. When we refer to the feet or legs being 'hip-width apart' this is what we mean.

Stabilizing the Pelvis

- Use the mirror in profile.
- Place your hands over your lower abdominals. Take a breath in and feel the abdominals rise under your hands.
- Breathe out and think of pressing the air out slowly from the lower abdominals. As you expel the last atom of breath you should feel them hollowing and firming up under your hands. This deep abdominal muscle is 4 layers down so you might need to press down with the fingers a little to feel the contraction or engagement.
- You do not have to be breathing out to find this muscle. Imagine doing up a tight pair of jeans when you have to pull in the lower abdominals so as not to catch your skin in the zip. It is not the same as pulling in the waist when doing up a tight belt. Practise them both and try to isolate the in-pull between the navel and the pubic bone. The pelvis does not move!
- If you have trouble feeling this hollowing try the following: turn over on to all fours, place a mirror at your side or under your abdomen and pull your shirt or leotard up to reveal your stomach. Breathe in and note how the lower abdominals drop towards the floor. Breathe out and slowly draw them in, as if forcing the air out from between the navel and the pubic bone. Do 3 breaths, releasing the abdominals on the 'in' breath and drawing them up to the spine on the 'out' breath. Look in the mirror to check for unwanted movement in the pelvis or the spine. The only movement you should see is the lower abdominals closing up towards the spine. Your ribs will also close a little, but you should not feel the upper abdominals contract.
- Now breathe in and out without letting the lower abdominals drop at all. Your breath must go into the ribcage. Think of expanding the lower ribs into the back. In this four-point-kneeling position your ribs are really free to move.
- Practise the hollowing and back breathing in the Relaxation Position. Place the hands on the lower abdominals so you can feel for unwanted movement.

The Pelvic Floor

If you still cannot find this deep abdominal muscle, the other thing to try is a pelvic floor contraction.

The best way to recruit the pelvic floor muscles is, as you breathe out, to think of closing the sphincters that stop urine flow. Women can also imagine two doors sliding across the vaginal passage. Close them and then draw up, as if trying to suck a matchstick up inside, or think of water going down a plughole – except it's going up. Men should think of drawing their testicles up. Some men have success by imagining they are lifting a light weight with their penis as they close down the sphincters. The muscles used to stop you breaking wind can also help, but in my experience men seem to think 'better out than in' and have trouble finding this contraction! Do not use the buttocks. This is an unseen internal contraction and does not move the body. A pelvic floor contraction helps in drawing in the lower abdominals. The pelvic floor should always be engaged first, you then zip up and hollow the lower abdominals.

In the book I use many terms to describe how to stabilize the pelvis using the deep abdominal muscle, transversus abdominus and the pelvic floor but they all mean the same thing: scoop; hollow; draw the navel to the spine; suck in the lower abdominals; zip up and hollow.

This short warm-up has been devised to awaken your awareness of the deep abdominal muscle, transversus abdominus, the shoulder stabilizers and to lengthen the spine, all of which are important throughout the programme. You should always prepare your body for the mat programme, whichever version you are doing, with these few exercises.

The Warm-Up

Leg Slides

Aim
To stabilize the pelvis and lower back while moving a limb.

Starting Position
From the Relaxation Position (page 21), breathe out and engage the deep abdominals.

Note →

It is important for you to be able to keep the navel to spine and pelvic stabilization during the out and the in breath. You should not move on to the harder exercises until you can do this.

Movement
- Breathe in to prepare, keeping hollowed.
- Breathe out and slide the left leg away along the mat in line with the hip socket. The pelvis and spine should not move.
- Breathe in and hold.
- Breathe out, scoop out the abdominals without any movement in the pelvis, and drag the foot back along the floor towards your sit bones without any movement in the pelvis or back and without pressing the resting foot into the floor. The resting leg and hip are dissociated, relaxed.
- Breathe in and maintain your neutral spine and pelvis position.
- Breathe out and repeat with the right leg.
- Do 5 slides with each leg.

When proficient, change the breath control so you breathe out to slide the leg away and breathe in to slide it back.

Check Points
- Keep the resting leg relaxed and do not grip across the hip especially when dragging the foot back.
- Place your hands on the hip bones to check for unwanted movement.
- Keep the head, neck and chest relaxed and heavy on the mat.
- Check your leg is in line with the hip socket as it slides away. The knee points straight to the ceiling.

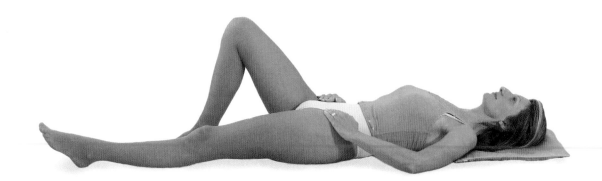

Spine Curls

Aim

To articulate and lengthen the spine and level the hips.
To improve the pelvic floor muscles and tone the buttocks
and the backs of the thighs.

Starting Position

Assume the Relaxation Position (page 21). Make sure your
feet are level.

Movement

- Breathe in to prepare, stretching the back of the ribs
  sideways on the mat.
- Breathe out and, engaging the pelvic floor and
  scooping out the lower abdominals, curl the tailbone
  up off the mat. Drop the waistline into the floor, pinning
  it there with your navel, like a mattress button, feeling
  the muscles in the lower back lengthen. Squeeze the
  buttocks, continuing to lift the vertebrae off the mat,
  one at a time until you are supported by your
  shoulders. **(1 to 4)**
- Breathe in and hold the position. The breath is in the
  ribcage. Do not allow your navel to come away from
  the spine. Maintain the pelvic curl. **(4)**
- Breathe out and, starting from the breastbone, start to
  lower each vertebrae back on to the mat. Channel your
  energy below the breastbone. Keep the shoulders
  relaxed into the mat and the head still. Lower the
  vertebrae back one at a time until the tailbone is on the
  mat and the pelvis and spine are in neutral again.
  (reverse 4 to 1)
- Do 6 to 8 repetitions.

Check Points

- Use the mirror in profile and check you are working
  through each vertebra and that your body is in a
  straight line from the shoulders to the knees in
  the bridge.
- Place your hands on your pelvis to check your hips
  stay level.
- Do not allow the knees to fall open or come together;
  they should remain hip-width apart.
- Focus your eyes in front of you on where the ceiling
  meets the wall and keep the head still. It might want
  to tip backwards.

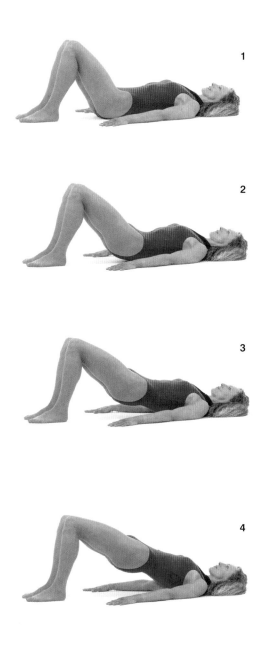

1

2

3

4

Hip Rolls

Aim
To stretch and rotate the spine.

Starting Position
From the Relaxation Position (page 21), bring the feet and knees together, connecting the inner thighs. You could place a tennis ball between the knees to keep them on a level plane. During the exercise knee stays over knee and ankle over ankle. Keep the tailbone down. Open the arms out to the sides; the hands should be a little lower than the level of the shoulders. Turn the palms up to the ceiling. This helps open the chest. **(1)**

Movement
- Breathe in to prepare, keeping navel to spine.
- Breathe out and, keeping the knees together, move the legs to the right and roll the head towards the left. Turn the left palm down as you move. The soles of the feet will come off the mat as you keep the inner borders of the feet together. Control the rotation in the spine allowing it to peel off the mat up to your shoulders which remain grounded. Your left ear should be on or near the mat. **(2)**
- Breathe in and hold the position. It is important not to release the lower abdominals as you breathe here.
- Breathe out and begin pulling the ribs and upper vertebrae back down into the mat. As you move, turn the left palm back up. The abdominals must work. Continue until the pelvis settles back into neutral and the knees are centred.
- Breathe in and hold.
- Breathe out and repeat the twist to the left, turning the head to the right.
- Do 6 to 8 repetitions alternating sides.

Check Points
- The knees are the first to move and the last to return.
- Do not tuck the pelvis under when returning. Keep in neutral.
- The arms, shoulders and neck stay relaxed and heavy on the mat.
- Keep the knees together or you will lose the stretch.
- Feel the feet heavy on the mat when you return to centre.
- Use the breathing to help in opening and closing the ribcage.

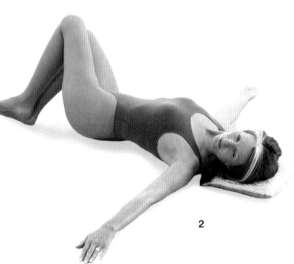

2

1

Single Knee Folds

Aim

To awaken the pelvic stabilizers and practise leg movement with pelvic stability. You will need to lift the legs on and off the mat throughout the programme using these Knee Folds. They are technical and need concentration even though they are ultimately only transitions to get you from one position to another.

Starting Position

Get into the Relaxation Position (page 21) and make sure your legs and feet are correctly aligned. Engage the deep pelvic stabilizers by hollowing the lower abdominals and drawing in the pelvic floor. **(1)**

Movement

- Breathe out and hinge the left leg up, lifting from the powerhouse, to bring the knee over the hip socket. Keep the tailbone long and heavy on the mat and the foot in a parallel line with the knee. Feel the thigh bone dropping down snugly into the hip socket. **(2)**
- Breathe in and hold the position.
- Breathe out and slowly lower the leg. To keep the pelvis and back still you must increase the work in the lower abdominals as the foot nears the floor.
- Breathe in and rest.
- Repeat with the right leg.
- Repeat the lifts 4 times on each leg.

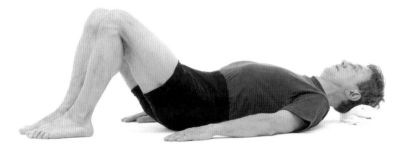

1

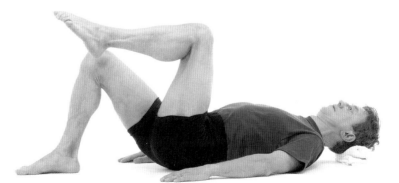

2

Double Knee Fold

Aim

To get both legs above the body without moving the spine or pelvis. You need more strength in the powerhouse to do this version.

Starting Position

As for Knee Folds (page 27).

Movement

- Breathe out and hinge the left leg up. **(1)**
- Breathe in and hold.
- Breathe out and hinge the right leg up to join the left. Connect the inner thighs and ankles. You are now in the Double Knee Fold position. **(2)**
- Breathe in and hold the position.
- Breathe out and slowly lower the left leg back down in line with the left sit bone.
- Breathe in and hold.
- Breathe out and lower the right leg down.
- Repeat, starting with the right leg.
- Do 4 Knee Folds alternating the leg you start with.

Check Points

- Keep the upper body relaxed. The spine must not arch off the mat so anchor it by keeping the ribcage and pelvis pressing into the mat.
- Keep the spine and pelvis in neutral.
- Place your hands on the lower abdominals to check they do not bulge upwards, especially on the second leg lift and the first leg descent.

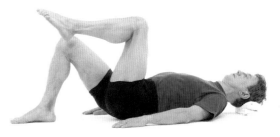

1

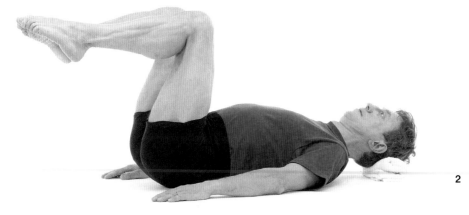

2

Abdominal Preparation

When performing an abdominal curl-up or sit-up, the tendency is for the head to lead the movement and to poke forward, straining the neck. Whenever you go to curl up through the spine you must start with the nodding movement we use to say 'yes'. The rotation axis is round the ears. Put your fingers in your ears and imagine a line through your head from ear to ear. Try nodding round this axis. Lift the head with the eye focus down and from then on the head stays still and the flexion comes from the breastbone. During the Pilates programme, there are many exercises that use the abdominals to curl up through the spine. Always remember to use this sequence. It will avoid unnecessary neck strain.

Use the mirror or ask a friend to check your head position in each exercise. The ears should remain in line with the shoulders and not in front of them.

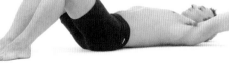

1

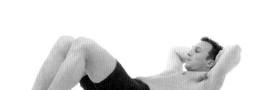

2

Curl-Ups

Aim
To train the muscles to move in the correct sequence (to pattern the body), to perform a curl-up without suffering tension in the neck and to isolate the spinal flexors without using the hip flexors.

Starting Position
Assume the Relaxation Position (page 21). Reach the arms away past the hips so you have a good gap between the ear and the collarbone. Keeping the gap between the ears and shoulders, clasp the hands behind the head. Have your elbows slightly forward so they are within your peripheral vision. Once you have gained this length in the neck, relax the back of the shoulders into the mat. This will help release the muscles over the top of the shoulders and allow the head and neck to curl up freely. **(1)**

Movement
- Breathe in to prepare. Hollow your navel to your spine.
- Breathe out as you drop the chin down, sliding the back of the skull up the mat a little. Look down towards your pelvis or even your breastbone.
- Peel your head and shoulders off the mat, breaking at the breastbone. Keep the chest open. Watch your pubic bone and make sure it does not tilt towards you. It will want to move, but you must use the deep abdominal stabilizers of the pelvis to keep the tailbone down on the mat. **(2)**
- Breathe in and hold the curl-up, keeping navel to spine.
- Breathe out and peel back down again, releasing from the breastbone and resting the head down last. Keep the elbows within the peripheral vision.
- Do up to 10 repetitions.

Check Points
- Do not poke the head forward. Your ears stay in line with the shoulders or even slightly behind them with the chin down.
- Keep your focus down.
- Maintain an open chest, keeping the elbows open.
- The legs remain relaxed with your weight resting evenly on the feet.

Shoulder Shrugs

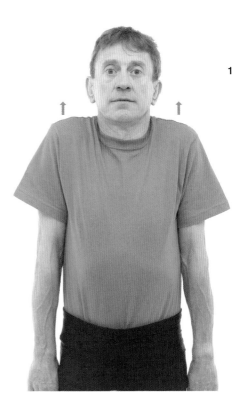

1

Aim
To find the muscles which hold the shoulders down and to practise keeping an open chest before performing the One Hundred on page 34.

Starting Position
Lie on the mat in the Relaxation Position (page 21) with your arms by your sides and the palms facing down. Keep a small gap between the arm and the body by the armpit. The elbows are softly rounded.

Movement
- Breathe in and shrug the shoulders right up to your ears. **(1)**
- Breathe out and slowly draw the collarbones away from the ears, keeping the entire back of the arm on the mat and reaching the fingers away to the feet. As you get to the depth of the movement you should feel a gentle stretch from the back of the ear to the collarbone and the back of the arm will want to roll forward off the mat. Don't let it. You should have a feeling of openness across the chest. **(2)**
- Do 8 shrugs.

Check Points
- Do not allow the chest to pop up as you reach down to the feet.
- Keep the back of the neck long on the mat.
- Do not squeeze the arms in towards the armpits. Keep the elbows soft. The work is round the back of the shoulder blade.

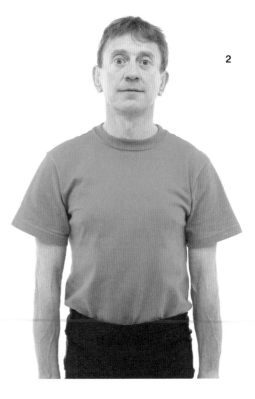

2

'I SPENT MY SCHOOL DAYS
AVOIDING ANYTHING THAT
MADE ME BREATHLESS AND
SWEATY AND NOW I AM THE
ONLY GIRL I KNOW WHO
HAS NEVER BELONGED TO A
GYM, LET ALONE SET FOOT
ON A RUNNING MACHINE.
THE ONLY REASON MY BODY
KEEPS FUNCTIONING IS
BECAUSE OF PILATES. I REALLY
DO IT TO GET AWAY FROM
THE TELEPHONE. BUT SOME-
HOW IF YOU CONCENTRATE
AND OBEY THE MASTER,
ENGAGE YOUR PELVIC FLOOR,
DO DOUBLE LEG STRETCHES
AND RESIST THE SPRINGS ON
THE REFORMER, YOUR BODY
LENGTHENS, STRENGTHENS
AND GETS MORE FLEXIBLE.
YOUR POSTURE IMPROVES,
YOUR MIND CLEARS AND
YOU CAN EAT MORE.'

NICOLA FORMBY,
'THE BLONDE' JOURNALIST

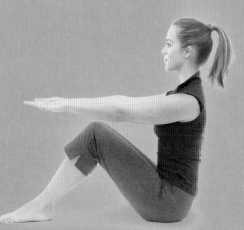

The Programme

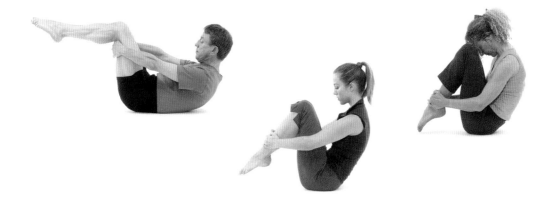

After the warm-up, you must start with the essential exercises at beginners' level. Once you've become proficient with these exercises, move on to the rest of the beginners' programme, adding the exercises in the order they are presented in the book.

Once you're confident with the beginners' programme, start to introduce the intermediate versions of the exercises into your workout. If you find any exercise particularly difficult, stay with the beginners' version until you are strong enough or flexible enough to move on.

Similarly, do not try the advanced versions of the exercises until you are confident you can do the intermediate version with ease and grace. Again, you may find you need to stay with some of the intermediate versions of some exercises for longer while moving on to the advanced versions for other exercises. Always work within your own level.

The One Hundred

Warning

If you have a neck problem, for example whip lash,
you might find the muscles in the neck tire easily. Pop
a hand under the back of the skull and swap hands
halfway through.

Be careful not to go to the intermediate or advanced
positions too quickly if you have back problems. You must
gain abdominal strength before lowering the legs.

Aim

To warm the body, alert the powerhouse and strengthen
the abdominals. To force you to breathe into the back
of the ribs.

The One Hundred

Starting Position

You will have finished the Warm-Up with the Shoulder Shrugs (page 30), which are meant to stabilize the shoulders before you start. From the Relaxation Position (page 21), do a Double Knee Fold (page 28). The feet are softly pointed. Connect the inner thighs and hollow your navel to your spine.

Movement

- Breathe out and curl the head and shoulders off the mat, breaking from the breastbone. **(1)**
- Breathe in and keep the lower abdominals hollowed and reach away with the hands. Your eye focus should be down on your pelvic area.
- Breathe out and beat the arms up and down 5 times.
- Breathe in and beat the arms 5 more times. At first you might only be able to breathe in for 2 or 3 beats maintaining navel to spine. Work up to 5.
- Continue for another 20 beats.
- As you improve, you work up to beating 100 times, breathing in for 5 beats and out for 5.
- The beats are rapid. They are helping to warm up the body and pump the blood. The hands move up and down over a distance of approximately 15 cms. Think of using the backs of the arms and keep reaching away past the hips. Do not squeeze up by the armpits but leave a little window to help keep the chest open.

Check Points

- Keep the pelvis in neutral but think of pressing the spine, right down to the tailbone, into the mat. You should have a very small gap between your spine and the mat just above the crest of the hips. If you cannot keep the rest of the spine flat on the mat then bring the legs in towards you a little so you can press the ribs into the mat.
- Keep your focus down.
- Do not poke the head forwards in front of the shoulders. Shoulders stay coiled down the back. Think of lengthening the back of the skull directly away from the tailbone but remaining in the curl-up.
- Keep the inner thighs connected.
- Expand the ribs in the back as you breathe in.
- Do not let the lower abdominals rise on the in breath. You can use the mirror in profile to check you have not got a great gap between the spine and the mat and to check your head position – your ears should be behind the shoulders. Once you've checked remember to return the head to look at the abdominals.

Go to the Roll-Up on page 39. ➡

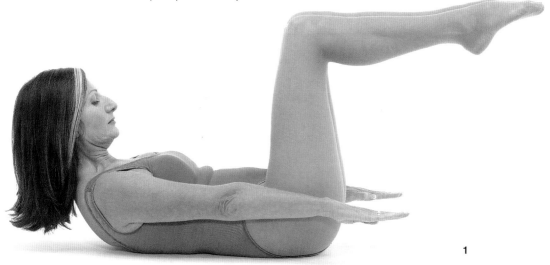

1

The One Hundred

This version puts a greater load on the pelvic stabilizers and the other abdominals. It also works the thighs.

Starting Position
As for beginners but the legs are extended.

Movement
- Breathe out and, as you curl the head and shoulders off the mat, hollow navel to spine and extend the legs keeping the inner thighs together. Softly point the toes. **(1)**
- Breathe in, beat the arms 5 times as for beginners, breathe out and beat the arms another 5 times. Continue until you have counted up to 100.
- Finish as for beginners.

Check Points
As for beginners but also:
- Your spine is more likely to lift from the mat so extra vigilance is needed to keep it pressed to the mat by using the abdominals.
- Keep the legs straight, sending energy right through them from the hip sockets and buttocks to the toes.

Go to the Roll-Up on page 40.

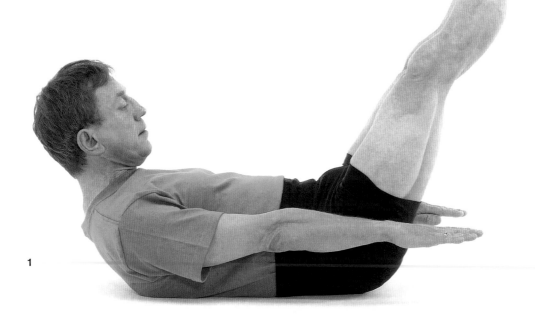

1

The One Hundred

This is the full version and requires a good deal of abdominal strength. It is very important to keep the spine pressed to the mat.

Starting Position
- As for beginners, but hinge the knees up over the chest so they are directly over the hips with the feet together. Then, open the knees shoulder-width apart keeping the feet in contact.
- Breathe out and curl the head and shoulders off the mat as you extend the legs. The knees are rotated slightly outwards and the inner thighs are connected. Think of wrapping the buttocks round from beneath and feel the backs of the legs supporting the thighs. **(1)**

Movement
- Breathe in and breathe out beating the arms as for the intermediate version.
- Count 20 breaths (100 beats).
- Finish as for beginners, breathing in to bring the knees in towards the chest, and out to roll back down through the spine.

Check Points
- Keep the abdominals scooped and the navel pinned into the spine.
- Press the back of the spine to the mat.
- Keep the tailbone down and the back of the skull lengthened away from it.
- Keep the shoulders drawn down the back.
- Squeeze the buttocks together and feel them and the backs of the thighs supporting the legs.
- Keep the tops of the inner thighs squeezed together.
- Break from the breastbone.

Go to the Roll-Up on page 42. ➡

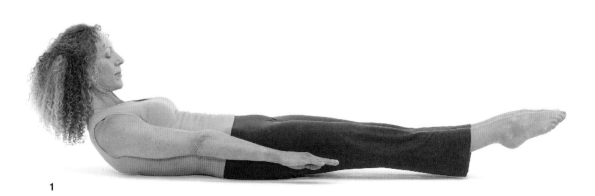

1

The Roll-Up

Warning

Not suitable for people with spinal disc problems.

Aim

To articulate the spine, stretching out tight areas.

To strengthen the abdominals.

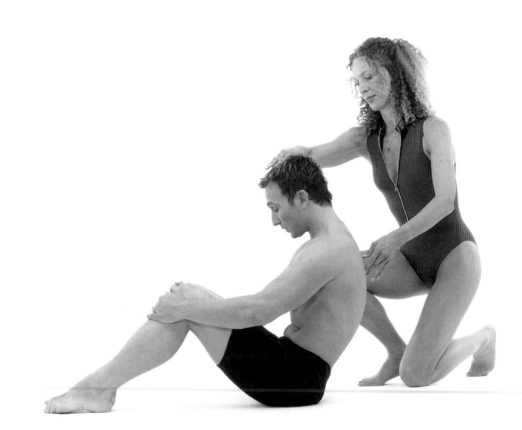

The Roll-Up

Starting Position
Sit up with the knees bent, the feet hip-width apart
and the hands round the outside of the knees. Adjust
the feet so that you can sit up with a flat back.

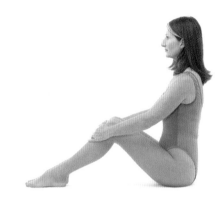

1

Movement
- Breathe in and sit up tall out of the hips. Think of sliding
  the back up a pole or a wall. Round the elbows to help
  open the chest and keep a gap between the shoulders
  and the ears. Focus straight ahead. **(1)**
- Breathe out and drop your eye focus down to your pelvis
  as you hollow the lower abdominals and rotate the pelvis
  forward under you, using the lower abdominals. Think of
  pulling the mat under you with the sit bones. Roll the
  base of the spine and the pelvis down on the mat,
  allowing the hands to slide down the thighs. **(2)**
- When you feel your legs want to straighten, the feet
  want to lift, or you feel you are going to collapse down,
  stop. **(3)**
- Breathe in and hold the position. Breathe into the back
  of the ribs and keep the abdominals scooped inwards.
- Breathe out as you slowly roll back up keeping your
  focus down on your abdominals. You must not hinge up
  from the hips, but roll up over the waistline, breaking
  from the breastbone and leading with the crown of the
  head. **(reverse 3 to 1)**
- Breathe in. Once the shoulders are right over the hips,
  you re-stack the spine to assume the starting position
  looking straight ahead.
- Do 6 repetitions.

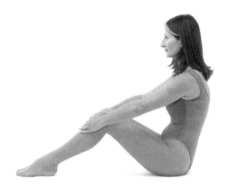

2

Check Points
- As you roll backwards, try and relax the muscles at the
  front of your hips, which join the legs to the pelvis.
- Keep the chest soft and open and the shoulders down
  the back.
- As you roll back up, start from the breastbone and not
  from the front of the hips.
- Keep the soles of the feet flat on the floor and the
  second toes in line with the knees.
- Do not hold your breath.
- Relax the hands and arms.

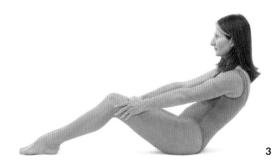

3

Go to Single Leg Circles on page 49. ▦▦▶

The Roll-Up

This requires more abdominal strength and articulates the whole spine.

Transition and Starting Position

From the end of the One Hundred (page 36), Double Knee Fold down using the correct technique described on page 28. The feet are together, the knees bent enough to have the soles of the feet on the mat and the inner thighs are connected. Simultaneously, place both arms down alongside your body on the mat and reach away towards your feet. **(1)**

Movement

- Breathe in to prepare, drawing the breath into the ribs and hollowing the abdominals.
- Breathe out and peel the head, shoulders and the rest of the spine slowly off the mat, one vertebra at a time. Slide the hands along the mat to help the spine articulate and to keep the chest open. **(2 to 4)**
- Breathe in when the shoulders are over the hips, before you re-stack the spine to assume the starting position, and sit up with a straight back. The arms are parallel and raised in front of you at shoulder height. **(5)**
- Breathe out and tuck the pelvis under to start slowly rolling the spine back down on to the mat, one vertebra at a time. Watch your alignment. Roll in a straight line. Your head will settle last as you finish the out breath. **(reverse 5 to 1)**
- Breathe in and start the roll-up again.
- Repeat 6 to 8 times.

Check Points

- Do not hinge from the hips. Roll smoothly through each segment of your back.
- Keep the head at the end of the spine when rolling down. It will tend to poke forward.
- Do not allow the abdominals to bulge.
- When rolling up, try to keep the tailbone down as you slide the ribs down towards the pelvis.
- Use your stomach muscles to isolate each vertebra.
- Do not hunch the shoulders. Try to keep the chest open and relaxed.

Go to the Roll Over on page 45.

1

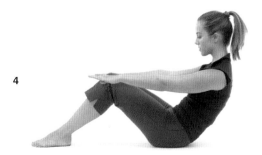

2

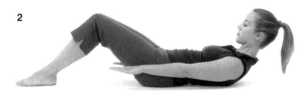

3

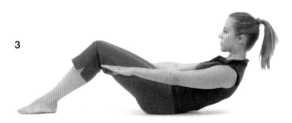

5

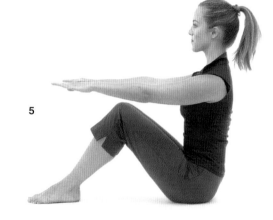

4

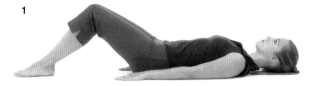

The Roll-Up

If you can roll up with the legs bent, as in the intermediate version, you are safe to roll up with straight legs. This version also stretches the spine as well as articulating the vertebrae and strengthening the abdominals.

Transition and Starting Position

From the end of the One Hundred (page 37), Double Knee Fold (page 28) down squeezing the knees together. Breathe in to prepare, then breathe out and extend the legs along the mat and, simultaneously, roll down through the spine and place the arms above your head on the mat. Close the ribs down and hollow the abdominals. Squeeze the inner thighs and the buttocks, without tipping the pelvis out of neutral. Flex the feet. **(1)**

Movement

- Breathe in and begin to lift the arms over your body. When they are above your chest, peel the head off the mat, first tucking the chin down, and start to roll up through the spine. **(2)**
- Breathe out as you reach the most difficult part of the roll-up when the tips of the shoulder blades down to the lower back come up off the mat vertebra by vertebra. **(2 to 3)**
- Keep exhaling as you hold the curve of the spine with the pelvis tucked under you and reach forward with the hands towards the toes. **(4)**
- Breathe in as you start to roll back down, initiating the movement from the sit bones, making sure your shoulders stay down the back and your head is at the end of your spine. **(5)**
- Breathe out as you roll through the upper back and release the shoulders, head and arms back down on the mat, with the arms above the head. The out breath will leave the ribs closed down and the abdominals scooped out ready for the next roll-up. **(6 to 7)**
- Do 6 to 8 repetitions. Stop if you start to lose the technique. Do just 3 good repetitions if necessary.

Check Points

- It is very important to roll smoothly through the spine, especially in the lower back. Keep a flowing pace. The whole roll-up moves at the same speed.
- Keep the abdominals scooped.
- Push through the heels.
- Do not hunch the shoulders. Keep the chest soft and open.
- Look down through the roll-up.
- Keep the buttocks squeezed and the inner thighs connected.

Go to the Roll Over on page 46. ➡

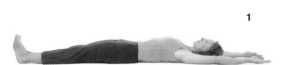

1

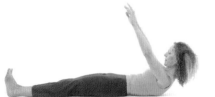

2

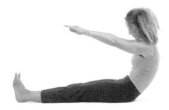

3

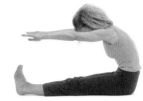

4

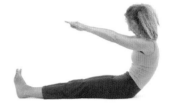

5

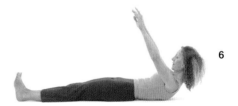

6

7

The Roll Over

Warning

Be careful if you have neck problems. Read the instructions fully before deciding whether or not to attempt the exercise. It is also not suitable if you have disc problems.

Aim

To stretch the spine and the backs of the legs and to strengthen the powerhouse. The emphasis is on a steady flow of movement as you isolate each vertebra both on the roll over and on the roll back.

The Roll Over

Transition and Starting Position

Remove your head support. From the last Roll-Up (page 40), bend the knees in towards the chest, remembering to keep the pelvis still and the abdominals hollowed, and then lift the legs up above the hips with the inner thighs connected. At this stage, you keep the knees half bent. Softly point the feet. Open the arms into a low 'V' along the floor. **(1)**

Movement

- Breathe in and slowly bring the legs over the body, keeping the tailbone down and lengthened away. **(2)**
- Breathe out and curl the tailbone and spine off the mat, pressing down gently into the floor with the arms and using the abdominals. **(3)**
- Keep the neck long, anchoring the back of the skull on the mat. Continue to roll the spine off the mat, making sure your hips are square and your legs are directly over the body. The toes are aiming for the floor behind your head. Do not roll so far that you feel pressure on the head and neck. You should be able to lift the head.
- Breathe in and open the legs a little wider than the shoulders. **(4)**
- Breathe out and, with great control, roll the spine back down on to the mat using the abdominals to control the movement. Keep the back of the neck long and the backs of the shoulders and arms flat on the floor. **(reverse 4 to 1)**
- Keep breathing out as you bring the legs back up over the hips and close them together, releasing the tailbone to the mat. Your upper back should be firm to the mat along with the pelvis as you return to neutral spine and pelvis.
- Do 3 roll overs and then reverse, starting with the legs in the open position and then closing them together as you roll back.
- Use the same breathing pattern.

Check Points

- This movement is performed at a steady pace. No acceleration or deceleration.
- As you roll the spine up, use the lower abdominals to start and then feel the upper abdominals working by the ribs to get the upper back off the mat.
- Keep the chest open and the arms reaching down past the hips.
- Keep the head still, it will want to tip upwards.
- Do not let the knees turn inwards. Even though the legs are bent you can still maintain proper leg alignment. See technique on page 50.

Go to Single Leg Circles on page 50.

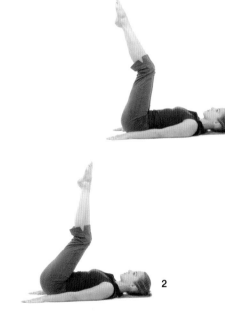

1

2

3

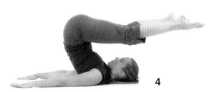

4

The Roll Over

Transition and Starting Position

Remove your head support. From the end of the last Roll-Up (page 42), bend the knees in towards the body and straighten them above the hips with the inner thighs connected and the feet softly pointed. Open the arms along the mat to a low 'V'. Keeping the upper back firmly on the mat and the spine and pelvis in neutral, lower the legs slightly towards the floor. You must not let the back arch, so only lower as far as you are able. **(1)**

Movement

- Breathe in and start to hinge the legs over your body, lengthening through the sit bones. **(2)**
- Breathe out and, when your hips start to lift, use the lower abdominals to curl the spine off the mat, keeping the legs straight and aiming the feet at the floor behind you. **(3)**
- Breathe in and open the legs to shoulder-width apart. Keep the navel to the spine. **(4)**
- Breathe out and, with control, roll the spine back on to the mat, lowering it with your abdominals. Keep the knees straight and the toes pushing away.
- Keep breathing out as you lower the tailbone on to the mat and bring the legs back to the starting position. Keep the back down and the abdominals flat! **(reverse 4 to 1)**
- Do this 3 times and then reverse, starting with the legs open and closing them when rolled back on the shoulders.

Check Points

As for intermediate but also:

- The legs will want to bend, don't let them. You should feel a slight stretch in the back of the thighs.
- Keep the pelvis square.
- Keep the legs on the same level. One might end up closer to your body than the other. Watch them.

Go to Single Leg Circles on page 52. ⟹

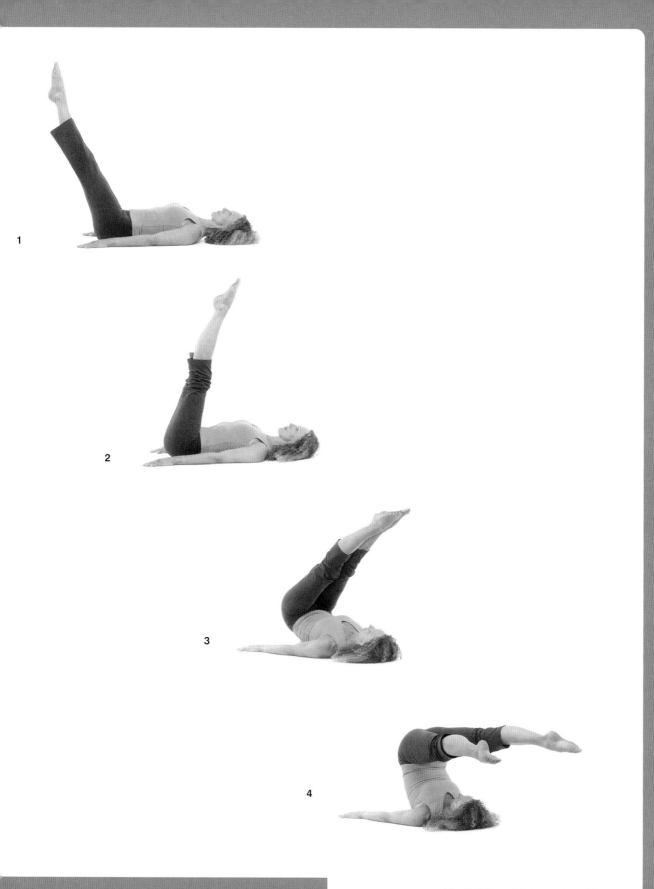

1

2

3

4

Single Leg Circles

Warning

If you suffer from arthritis in the hip, keep the circles fairly small and within a comfortable range.

Aim

To mobilize the hips and strengthen the thighs and the deep abdominals.

Single Leg Circles

Starting Position

From the Relaxation Position (page 21) **(1)**, zip up and hollow the lower abdominals and, breathing out, bring your right leg up in a Single Knee Fold (page 27) so the knee is over the hip socket and the foot is in line with the knee. The arms are in a low 'V' at your sides but while you are learning it is a good idea to place your fingertips on your hip bones so you can be sure they remain still. Keep the resting leg bent on the floor and do not press down on it during the circles, that's cheating!

Movement

- Breathe in and start to circle your thigh bone anti-clockwise from 12 o'clock round to 9 o'clock. **(2)**
- Breathe out and finish the remaining three-quarters of the circle back up to 12 o'clock. Imagine the action being like a pestle grinding something in a mortar. The head of the thigh bone revolves in the stable hip socket as the knee moves. Keep zipping and hollowing, especially at 6 o'clock and 3 o'clock, when the pelvis is most likely to tilt. Concentrate on relaxing the resting leg and hip joint and on the breathing. Use a short in breath and a longer and complete out breath.
- Do 5 circles and then reverse so you are going clockwise for another 5.
- To finish, breathe in to prepare, keeping navel to spine, and out to place the foot back on the floor in the Relaxation Position.
- Repeat the exercise with the other leg.

Check Points

- Single Leg Circles involve a good deal of core stability. Use the zip up and hollow throughout.
- The entire upper body remains relaxed, especially the head and shoulders. If the trunk lifts or rolls with the movement, try closing the ribs down to help ground this part of the spine.
- Keep the resting leg dissociated in the Relaxation Position with the knee in line with the hip socket and the second toe.
- The chest remains open and heavy to the floor.
- When you go to the 'V' position of the arms, try not to push down on them. The work is in the pelvic stabilizers.
- The foot is softly pointed and only moves with the thigh. Do not draw round the clock with it, draw with the thigh bone.
- Start and finish the circles with the knee opposite the hip socket. See leg alignment on page 17.

Go to Rolling Like a Ball on page 55. ▬▬▶

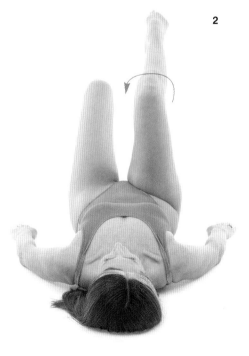

2

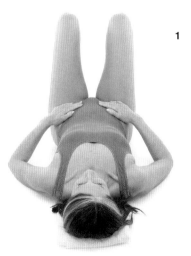

1

Single Leg Circles

Once you have gained the strength to hold the pelvis in neutral with the knee bent, you then straighten it out at an angle away from the body.

Transition and Starting Position
From the last Roll Over (page 45), bend and hinge the left leg down placing the foot on the mat opposite the sit bone with the knee bent. Making sure you keep zipped up and hollowed, stretch the right leg out. Keep the arms in a low 'V'. Keep the tailbone down.

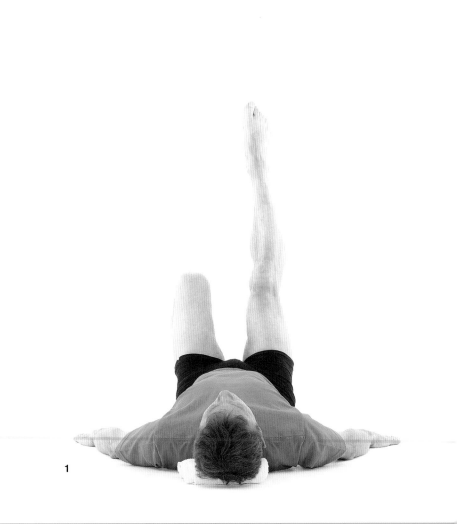

1

Movement

- Draw a circle anti-clockwise, as for beginners. Think of drawing round the clock with the toes rather than the knee. The movement is the same in the hip socket but the lever is longer with a straight leg and therefore the work to stabilize the pelvis is greater. **(1 to 3)**
- Use the same breathing as for the beginners' version.
- Do 5 circles in each direction and then change legs.

Check Points

As for beginners but also:

- Feel the energy coming out of the centre and down the leg to the top of the foot. You should feel the work in the thigh muscles.
- Bend the knee in a little if you cannot keep the pelvis in neutral or if you feel you are gripping in the hip socket.
- Be sure not to stabilize with the resting leg. Concentrate and breathe!

Go to Rolling Like a Ball on page 56.

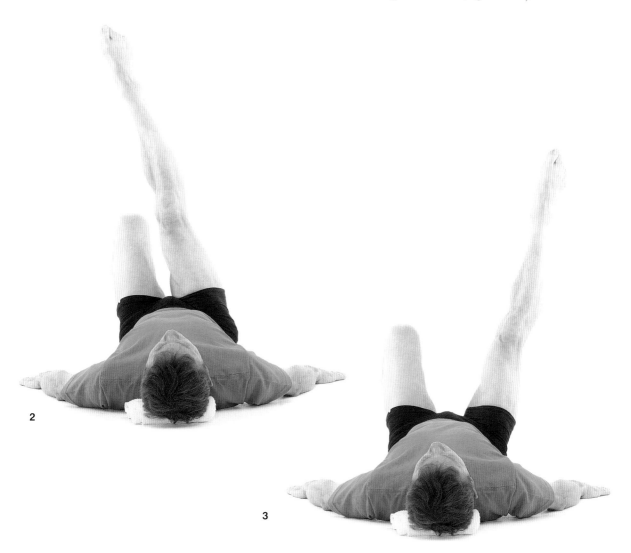

2

3

Single Leg Circles

Demands greater flexibility in the back
of the leg and strong thigh muscles.

Transition and Starting Position
From the last Roll Over (page 46), leave the right leg
extended above the hip or as close as you can to your
body without the tailbone rising from the mat. Breathe out
and, keeping a strong centre, lower the left leg to the mat,
in line with the hip. Flex the foot so the sole faces straight
ahead. Imagine it pressing flat against a wall.

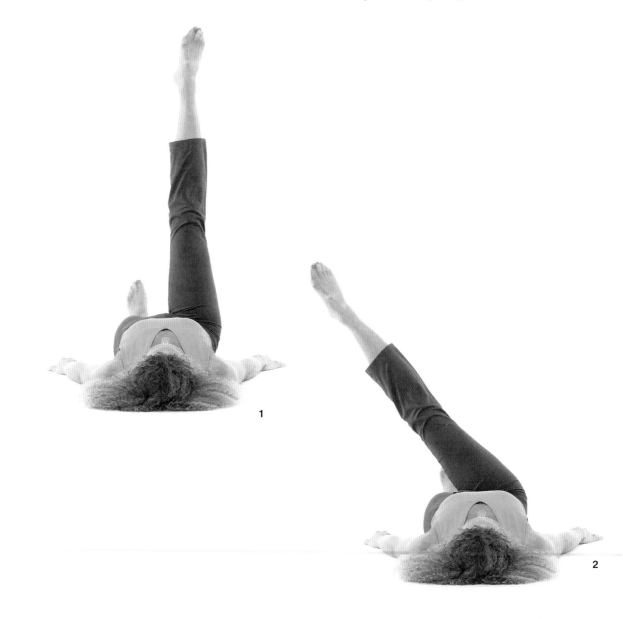

1

2

Movement

- As for beginners and intermediate: draw round the clock face anti-clockwise for 5 circles then clockwise for 5. **(1 to 4)**
- To change legs, breathe in to bend the knee in towards the chest and breathe out to slide it along the floor in line with the hip socket. Flex the foot.
- Breathe in and bend the left leg in towards the chest.
- Breathe out to stretch the leg up to the ceiling.

Check Points

As for beginners and intermediate but also:

- To help keep the pelvis still, and ground the hip and the back of the resting leg without tilting the pelvis.
- Keep both feet in good alignment (see leg alignment on page 17). The flexed foot on the resting leg has a mind of its own! Sit up and have a look at it before you start this advanced version for the first time.
- Make sure the hips stay square and the tailbone down on the mat.
- Keep a heavy chest and the upper back still.
- Let the head of the thigh bone drop into the hip socket of the working leg and then reach the toes to the ceiling and stretch the knee.
- Eye focus is straight up but if your chin tends to tip up, then focus on the knee.

Go to Rolling Like a Ball on page 57. ➡

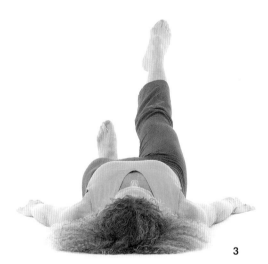

3

4

Rolling Like a Ball

Warning

Be careful if you have a neck problem which refers pain
into the arm. You must keep the chest open, the shoulders
down the back, and the head and neck relaxed.

Aim

To massage the spine and strengthen the abdominals.
You make the shape and then maintain it throughout.
In this exercise you find your centre of gravity through
balance.

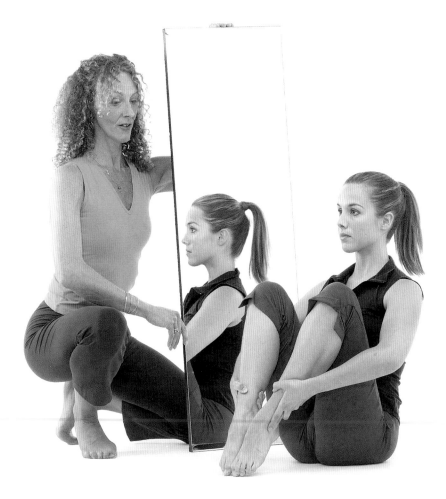

Rolling Like a Ball

Starting Position

Double Knee Fold (page 28) and connect the inner thighs. Hold the index and middle fingers of your right hand with the left hand behind the backs of the thighs. Peel your head and shoulders off the mat as you hollow your abdominals and pull the legs away from you. Keep the shoulders still and the chest open; the pull of the legs should not affect them. Look down. Press the lower spine and your waistline into the mat. **(1)**

Movement

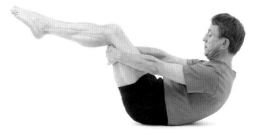

1

- Breathe out and rock slightly forward by pushing the legs into the hands. The knees remain bent and the lower legs are relaxed down by the buttocks. The inner thighs are connected. **(2)**
- Keep the rocker shape you are in and allow yourself to rock back. Use the abdominals to continue the small rock to and fro breathing normally from now on. Do not let the legs come in and out, they remain pushed away to form a stable rocker. It is the abdominals which do the work to keep the momentum of the first push.
- The rock is only small, rolling through the lower back where the pelvis meets the spine.
- Do up to 20 rocks to and fro. Rest and then repeat.
- If your arms are too short to get an open angle at the hip in the starting position, take a short pole, a belt, or a tie and hold it with the hands a few centimetres apart, behind the thighs. This will provide a little more length.

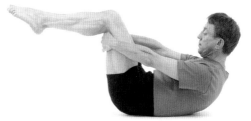

2

Check Points

- Try to keep the chin down, but the ears behind the shoulder line.
- Keep the tension of the legs pushing away. The angle between your thighs and hips remains constant.
- Concentrate all the time on keeping the shoulders down the back.
- Keep the abdominals hollowed.
- Make the shape and maintain it.
- Breathe normally.

Go to the Single Leg Stretch on page 59. ➡

Rolling Like a Ball

This version demands more work from the upper abdominals and a more flexible spine.

Transition and Starting Position

From the last Single Leg Circle (page 51), place the feet together on the mat a little further away from your sit bones than for the Relaxation Position (page 21). Connect the inner thighs and roll up through the spine so you are sitting up, keeping zipped and hollowed. Place your right hand round the right ankle and the left hand round the left ankle. Bring the knees slightly further in towards the chest. Hollow the abdominals and rock back on to the end of the spine. You should be at the front of the mat. Drop the chin and draw the shoulders down the back. Imagine you are curled up inside a huge beach ball. The toes are softly pointed and just off the floor.

Movement

- Breathe out and scoop out the abdominals, focusing down on your centre. **(1)**
- Breathe in and rock back using the abdominals. Roll through the spine smoothly and with control, on to the shoulders. The head stays tucked in and should not touch the floor behind you. **(2)**
- Breathe out and roll back up to the starting position without touching the floor with your toes or changing the roundness of the back. Stay in the ball shape.
- Repeat the roll up to 10 times with smooth control and following an imaginary straight line down the middle of the mat.
- The rhythm is like a pendulum with a milli-second pause at the end of the rock backwards and forward.

Check Points

- Keep in the round shape you made.
- Do not throw the head back, keep it tucked in and the focus down.
- Keep the heels the same distance from your bottom as when you started. They will want to pull away to achieve the movement. You must use your stomach muscles to move and to brake.
- Try not to hunch the shoulders, especially on the roll back up.
- Keep the abdominals pressing in towards the spine.
- Keep rolling in a straight line.

Go to the Single Leg Stretch on page 60. ➡

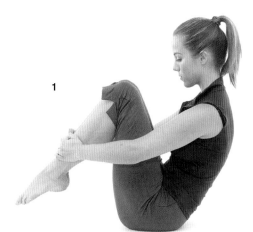

1

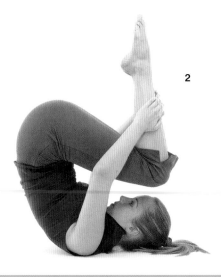

2

Rolling Like a Ball

Transition and Starting Position

From the last Single Leg Circle (page 53), lower the left leg straight down to the floor to join the other leg. Connect the inner thighs and flex the feet. Roll up through the spine as in the Roll Up (page 42). Stretch your body over your legs, keeping navel to spine, and place the hands round the ankles as described in the intermediate version. Roll up through the spine, gathering the legs into the chest, and rock back on to the tailbone. Bring the heels right in towards the buttocks and make a small ball. In this advanced version you make a much tighter ball. **(1)**

Movement

- As for the intermediate version. **(2)**
- Do up to 10 rolls.
- The smaller the ball, the harder it is on the abdominals to roll.

Check Points

As for intermediate version but even more effort is required to keep the tight shape and not to use the head or legs to achieve the roll.

Go to the Single Leg Stretch on page 61.

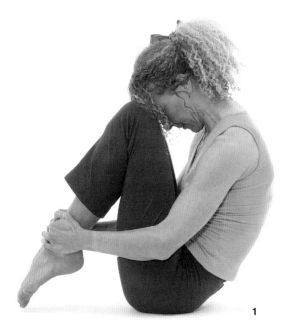

1

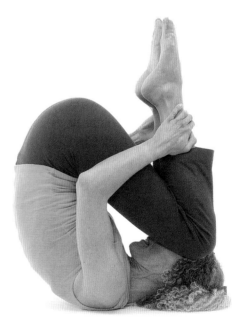

2

Single Leg Stretch

Aim

To open the lower back, stretch the leg and
work the abdominals with effort, coordination
and flowing movement.

Single Leg Stretch

Starting Position

From the Relaxation Position (page 21), Double Knee Fold (page 28) using the correct pelvic and spinal stabilization. Breathe out and curl the head and shoulders off the mat. Place your right hand over the front of your left knee. The hand comes from round the outside of the knee. Place the left hand, so it points towards the foot, along the left shin. Make sure the lower legs and feet are in alignment with the hip sockets. Scoop out the abdominals continuously. Your tailbone should remain lengthened along the mat with the pelvis in neutral.

Movement

- Breathe in to prepare.
- Breathe out and extend the right leg out and away from you in line with the hip, about 70–80 degrees above the floor, stretching through the knee joint but without snapping the joint into full extension. **(1)**
- Breathe in and bring the right leg back towards the chest. Swap the hand positions, reaching down the right shin with the right hand and placing the left hand over the left knee. Simultaneously extend the left leg away from you in line with the hip socket.
- The trunk should remain completely still, only the arms and the legs move.
- Keep the elbows open to help keep an open chest.
- Do 10 to 20 changes.
- To finish, breathe in and bring both knees in towards the chest, then breathe out to roll the head and shoulders back on to the mat.

Check Points

- When you breathe in, keep the navel pinned to the spine and the pelvis pressed to the mat.
- Keep the shoulders down and the chest open.
- Keep the head still and the focus down on the pelvis so you can watch for any unwanted movement.
- The toes are softly pointed throughout.
- Use the abdominals. Curl up off the mat from the breastbone and be careful not to lose the curl-up as you do the exercise.
- Do not poke the head forward. Remember, it is on the end of the spine so your ears are in line with the shoulders.
- The legs remain fairly high in this version to avoid straining the lower back.
- Do not snap the knee when extending the leg. Go smoothly into full extension. Think of controlling the movement by using the hamstrings in the back of the leg.

Go to the Double Leg Stretch on page 63. ➡

1

Single Leg Stretch

Transition and Starting Position

From the last Rolling Like a Ball (page 56), place the feet hip-width apart on the mat with the knees bent, and roll down through the spine into the Relaxation Position (page 21). Breathe out stretching the right leg out along the mat in line with the hip as you fold the left leg in towards the chest. Make sure your pelvis is square and you have the navel pinned into the spine. Place the hands as described in the beginners' version.

Movement

- Breathe in to prepare, keeping zipped and hollowed.
- Breathe out. Curl the head and shoulders up from the mat, simultaneously lifting the right leg off it up to about 45 degrees from the floor. Keep the pelvis still using your core stability. **(1)**
- Breathe in to change legs and continue as described for beginners. Your legs are slightly lower to the floor so the demand on the abdominals is increased in order to keep the pelvis in neutral.
- Use a little pressure from the hand over the knee to draw it down towards the chest without the tailbone lifting from the floor or twisting the pelvis.
- Do 10 to 20 changes.

Check Points

As for beginners but also:

- Only lower the legs to where you can keep zipped and hollowed.
- Keep the shoulders wide and down the back. The pulling of the knee to the chest demands greater attention to your shoulder stabilization.

Go to the Double Leg Stretch on page 64.

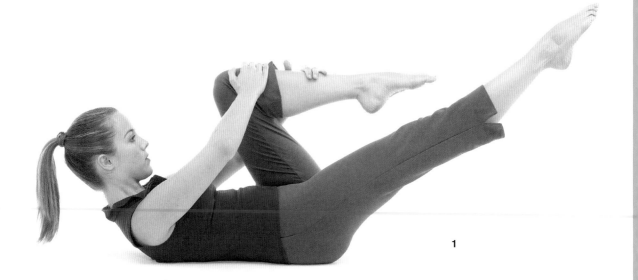

1

Single Leg Stretch

The legs are even lower here so the demand on core stability is even greater than in the intermediate version.

Transition and Starting Position

At the end of Rolling Like a Ball (page 57), you are balancing on the tailbone. Transfer the right hand over the left knee and the left hand to the left shin. Breathe out and, as you slowly extend the right leg out in line with the hip socket, roll down through the spine. Keep the eye focus on the pelvis and watch that it stays square. This is hard! The right leg is only a few centimetres from the floor. Squeeze the right buttock to help support the leg from beneath. **(1)**

Movement

- Breathe in as you change legs, extending the left leg away and squeezing the right knee into your chest.
- Breathe out and change legs again.
- Do a maximum of 24 changes, 12 on each leg.
- Once you have achieved this version and can maintain a strong, flat centre, change the breathing pattern so you breathe in for 2 leg stretches and out for 2.

Check Points

- As for the intermediate version but you must pay more attention to core stability and shoulder stabilization.
- When the leg is this low to the floor you should be able to feel the buttock on the outstretched leg working to help support from underneath.

Go to the Double Leg Stretch on page 65.

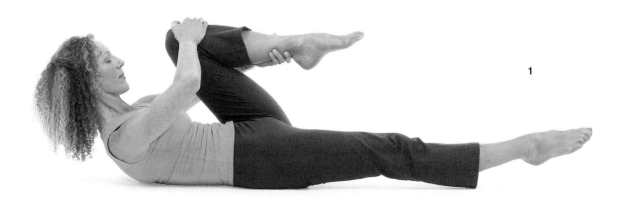

1

Double Leg Stretch

Warning
Be careful if you have back problems.

Aim
To work your powerhouse, the abdominals and the leg muscles. Everything flows out of a very strong centre.

Double Leg Stretch

Starting Position

From the Relaxation Position (page 21), Double Knee Fold (page 28) and connect the inner thighs. The toes are softly pointed and the tailbone is down on the mat. Breathe out and curl the head and shoulders off the mat. Reach your arms round the shins and hold them, easing them in towards your body. Keep the tailbone on the mat. If you are too stiff to bring the legs in together, separate the knees to hip-width apart but keep the feet together. When you extend the legs you must connect the inner thighs. This applies to all versions. **(1)**

Movement

- Breathe in to prepare and hollow navel to spine.
- Breathe out and straighten both your legs so they are at a slight angle to the floor. Keep the abdominals hollowed and think of pressing the spine to the mat without tilting the pelvis. Simultaneously extend your arms down the sides of the body with the palms facing down. Reach through the fingers, pulling the shoulders down the back. Keep your focus down on your centre and do not poke the head forward. **(2)**
- Breathe in and bend the knees back towards the chest.
- Bring the arms back and hug the legs to your chest. Have the elbows rounded to help open it.
- Keep lengthening through the tailbone remaining in neutral pelvis. Stay in the curl-up.
- Breathe out and repeat the movement.
- Do 6 repetitions.
- Once you have perfected this version change the breath control so you breathe in to straighten out the legs and breathe out to bring the knees back in and pump out the air from your lungs.
- To finish, roll the shoulders and head back on to the mat.

Check Points.

- Keep the chin down along with the eye focus.
- Do not allow the chest to close in as you reach down the body. Keep the inner thighs connected and the knees pointing straight towards you.
- Do not allow the abdominals to bulge away from the spine. Keep them hollowed.
- Think of the energy flowing out from your centre through the toes and the back of the skull.
- Keep the tailbone down throughout.
- Use the mirror in profile to check the back is not arching off the mat.

Go to Spine Stretch Forward on page 73.

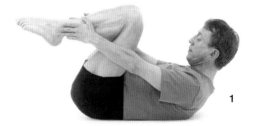

1

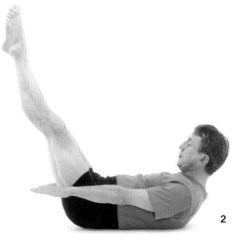

2

Double Leg Stretch

Once again, this version demands more core stability as the leverage of the legs is greater because they are lower and the arms also come into play.

Transition and Starting Position

From the last Single Leg Stretch (page 60), bend the knees in towards your body, and curl the head and shoulders back down to the mat. Change your hand positions so they are round the shins. Lengthen the tailbone to the floor. Breathe in to prepare then breathe out to curl the head and shoulders up off the mat. Look down. **(1)**

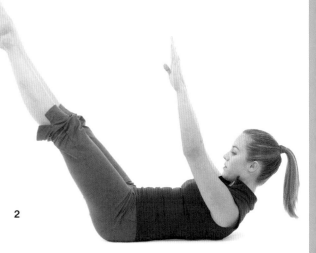

Movement

- Breathe in and, as you straighten your legs out and away from you, lift the arms straight up to above the shoulder joint. Do not let the body drop back, hold the curl-up and pin the navel to the spine. Breathe into the sides and back of the ribs and do not lose the upper back off the mat. Press down at the end of the breastbone. **(2)**
- Breathe out and circle the arms round, opening them to the sides and bringing them back in to gather your legs in towards the body. Pull the bent legs in to the chest. This stretches the lower back. Keep the pelvis in neutral, tailbone long. Do not lie down!
- Finish as for beginners.
- Do 6 repetitions.

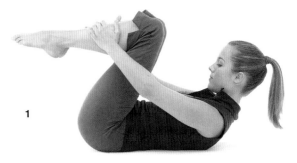

Check Points

- As for the beginners' version, but more effort will be needed to keep the back to the floor.
- Keep the focus down, especially during the arm lift.
- Keep the shoulders stabilized and an open chest. The arm movement might make you hunch. *Resist!*

Go to Straight Single Leg Raises on page 67. ➡

Double Leg Stretch

This should feel like a huge pump as the arms and legs extend away from a firm, flat centre.

Transition and Starting Position

Do not lie back down at the end of the last Single Leg Stretch (page 61). Breathe out and bend both knees in towards the body, grasping the legs round the shins. Check the pelvis is square. Your focus is down. **(1)**

Movement

- Breathe in and stretch the legs out and away from the centre as you lift the arms up with a straight back, so they are level with the ears. The arms should remain within your peripheral vision. The legs should be close to the floor. Only lower them as far as you can keep the back on the mat. **(2)**
- Breathe out and continue circling the arms, bending the knees back in towards the body. Squeeze out the air as you pull the legs in and keep lengthening through the tailbone. The pelvis stays still throughout.

Check Points

As for beginners' and intermediate versions but also:
- You are more likely to lose the curl-up when the arms are above the head. Emphasize the abdominal work under the breastbone and in the lower abdominals.
- Squeeze the lower buttocks to help stabilize the pelvis and support the legs during the extension.
- Keep the abdominals sucked into the spine!
- When drawing the legs back in, think of pulling them with your powerhouse.

Go to Straight Single Leg Raises on page 68. ➡

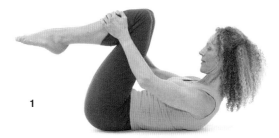

1

2

Straight Single Leg Raises

Aim

To work the leg muscles and stretch the backs of the
thighs. This exercise requires a very strong centre and
should be executed with precision and control. The
movement of the legs must not affect the pelvis!

Straight Single Leg Raises

Transition and Starting Position

From the last Double Leg Stretch (page 64), you roll the shoulders and head back down to the mat. Keep the legs folded over the body. Curl the head and shoulders back up to the curl-up position. Breathe out, scoop the abdominals, and stretch the left leg out in line with the hip socket a few inches off the mat. Hold the back of the right thigh and slightly straighten the right leg until you feel a gentle stretch up the back of it. Keep the tailbone down and the hips square. You should feel a slight stretch in the back of the thigh.

Movement
- Breathe in making sure you still have the navel pinned to the spine.
- Breathe out and pull the right thigh towards your chest with a controlled double pulse, 'in in'. Keep the sit bone and the tailbone lengthened into the mat. You will feel a gentle pull in the back of the thigh. Do not allow the leg to bend any more. **(1)**
- Breathe in and, with control, change legs, straightening the right leg out and away as you slightly bend the left leg and bring it in towards the body. The pelvis must not move. **(2)**
- Breathe out and holding the left thigh, repeat the double pulse.
- The feet remain in a soft point throughout.
- Continue, alternating legs, until you have done 5 repetitions with each leg.

Check Points
- The pelvis must stay still. Watch it!
- As you pulse the leg, keep the sit bone still; think of pressing it down towards the floor along with the tailbone.
- Do not hunch the shoulders.
- Keep the back of the skull lengthening away so as not to poke the head forward.
- The leg you are holding and pulsing towards your chest is slightly bent to allow you to keep the tailbone down and not take the stretch into the spine.

Go to Spine Stretch Forward on page 74. ➡

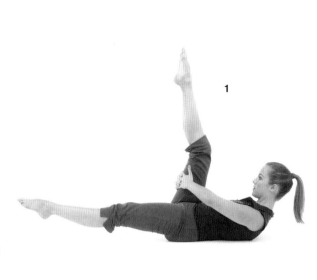

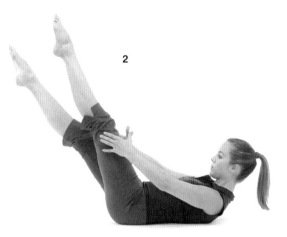

Straight Single Leg Raises

This version increases the flexibility in the backs of the legs because they must both stay straight.

Transition and Starting Position

Stay in the curl-up at the end of the last Double Leg Stretch (page 65), and extend the left leg out so it is just off the floor and in line with the hip. Simultaneously, hold the calf (or ankle if you are very flexible!) of the right leg as you straighten it out up to the ceiling in line with the hip. Check the hips stay square.

Movement

- As for intermediate.
- Do 5 repetitions on each leg.

Check Points

As for intermediate but also:

- The shoulders are more likely to hunch because you are reaching higher up the leg. Keep the chest open and the shoulders down.
- Apart from checking your leg alignment every now and then, the eye focus should stay down on the pelvis.
- The leg taking the stretch will be more likely to bend so keep stretching through the back of the knee.

Go to Straight Double Leg Raises on page 69.

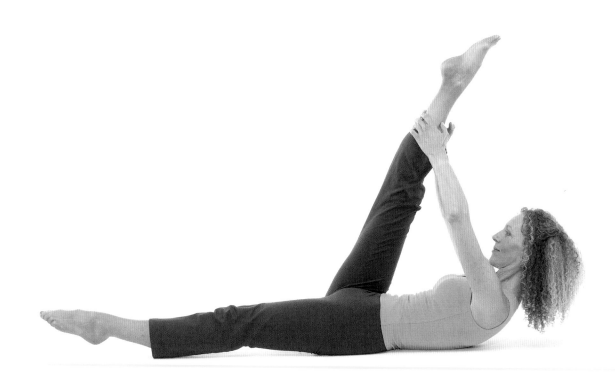

Spine Stretch Forward

Aim

To stretch the spine and allow you to really breathe.

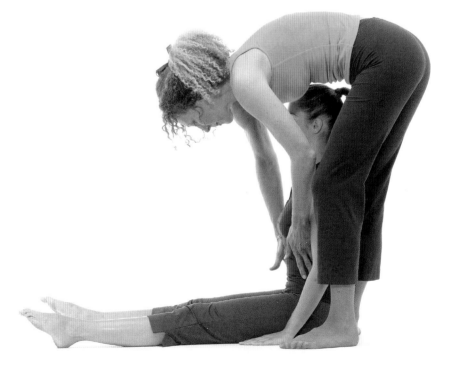

Check Points

- Open the left elbow behind you to help turn the body when you twist to the left and vice versa on the right. Do not think of pulling the other elbow forward towards the knee.
- Do not pull on the head. Keep the energy back into the hands.
- Turn round the spine and do not lose the curl-up.
- Hold the twist as you exhale all your air and reach back with the elbow.
- The leg extends and bends in line with the hip.

Go to Spine Stretch Forward on page 74.

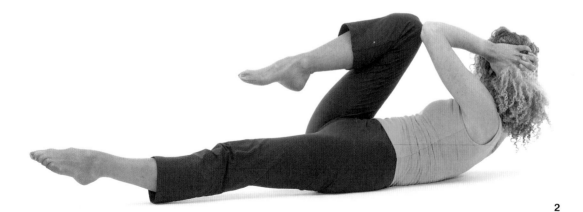

2

Criss-Cross

Aim

To work the oblique muscles of the abdominals and to rotate the spine.

Transition and Starting Position

From the last Straight Double Leg Raise (page 69), lower the left leg until it is just off the floor, simultaneously bending the right knee in towards the chest in line with the hip socket. The hands remain behind the head with the elbows open. Keep the pelvis square.

Movement

- Breathe out and turn the torso towards the left leg as you bring it in towards the chest bending it at the knee. Simultaneously extend the right leg out, just off the floor as you did in the Single Leg Stretch. **(1)**
- Breathe in to change legs and turn the torso towards the right knee as it comes in towards the chest. The pelvis remains anchored to the mat. **(2)**
- Do 10 changes.

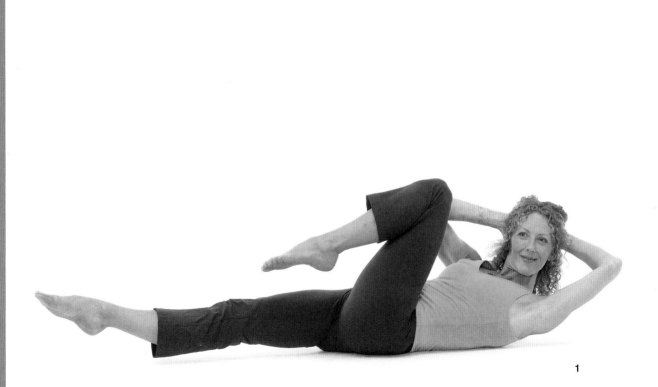

1

Straight Double Leg Raises

Warning
This will put a lot of stress on the lower back if not performed correctly.

Aim
To strengthen the abdominals and the big hip flexors. It needs great body awareness.

Transition and Starting Position
From the last Straight Single Leg Raise (page 68), bring the straight legs back together and connect the inner thighs. The legs are at right angles to the hip. You are still in the curl-up. Hold it! Rotate the legs from the hips outwards so the inner thighs remain connected but the knees are facing slightly outwards. They will form a small 'V' shape. The toes are softly pointed. Circle the hands and clasp them together round the base of the skull. Do not lose the curl-up. Keep the focus down.

Movement
- Breathe out and really hollow out the lower abdominals. They should be hollowed anyway! **(1)**
- Breathe in, making sure you breathe into the ribs and not into the abdominals, and slightly lower the legs towards the floor. Keep the pelvis still. Press the spine and tailbone down into the mat using your stomach muscles. **(2)**
- Breathe out and hinge the legs back up. Keep the tailbone on the floor! The pelvis should not move.
- Keep the movement small at first and increase the range as you gain strength.
- Build up to 6 repetitions.

Check Points
- The back must not arch.
- Use the inner thigh muscles and think of wrapping the buttocks round the backs of the legs and squeezing them to help support the weight of the legs as you lower. Use your pelvic floor muscles.
  - Break from the breastbone and hold the curl-up. Breathe!
  - The elbows are open and should be within your peripheral vision.
  - Draw the shoulders down the back.
  - Keep the chin down.
  - Do not let the abdominals bulge.

Go to Criss-Cross on page 70. ➡

1

2

Spine Stretch Forward

Starting Position

Sit up on the mat with the legs straight in front of you and about 2.5 centimetres wider apart than the shoulders. Look at your profile in the mirror and check your back is straight. If you cannot sit up straight and you are gripping in the hips, sit on a firm cushion or a telephone directory. A thick book is better because you will be able to feel your sit bones under you. Relax your feet, but make sure your knees are facing straight up. Place your hands by the outsides of your thighs. Imagine your spine running up the length of a wall or a pole. (This exercise can, in fact, be done against a wall.) Remember the tips of the ears should be in line with the shoulders and the shoulders directly over the hips.

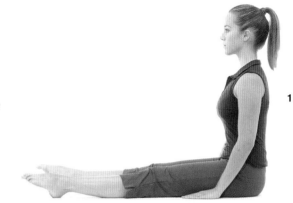

Movement

*   Breathe in, sitting up tall out of the hips and pinning your navel into the spine. **(1)**
*   Breathe out. Start by dropping the chin down, then slowly roll the spine off the imaginary pole or wall one vertebra at a time. As you roll forward slide the hands along the outer thighs. Do not let the shoulders hunch up, keep them down the back and the shoulder blades still on the ribs. **(2)**
*   At the depth of the stretch and the out breath, really pull your navel in and try and squeeze your buttocks.
*   Breathe in and out holding the stretch. Keep navel to spine. Feel the upper back stretch with the breath. **(3)**
*   Breathe out and slowly curl back up against the wall or imaginary pole, re-stacking the vertebrae one at a time. Keep the chest and shoulders relaxed and loose. **(reverse 3 to 1)**
*   Do up to 6 stretches.

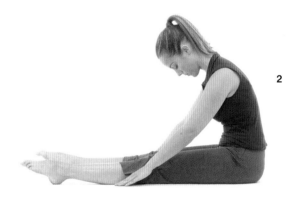

Check Points

*   The pelvis must stay still and not tip forward. Keep the sit bones grounded.
*   Lead the movement with the crown of the head.
*   Keep the shoulders away from the ears.
*   Do not grip in the fronts of the thighs.
*   The stretch is in the spine. You might feel a stretch in the backs of the legs as well if the muscles are very tight.

Go to the Saw on page 84. ➠

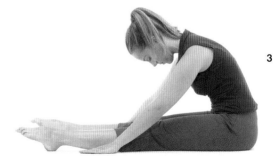

Spine Stretch Forward

This produces a greater stretch down the nerve paths and in the backs of the legs. Think of the body being like a huge breathing organism.

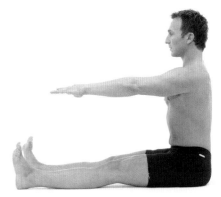

Intermediate Transition and Starting Position
From the last Straight Single Leg Raise (page 67), bend both knees back in towards your chest and hinge them, one at a time, back down on to the mat. Connect the inner thighs and place the arms alongside the body on the mat. Breathe out and roll up through the spine. Breathe in once the shoulders are over the hips and re-stack the spine so you are sitting up with a straight back. Stretch the legs out in front of you and open them so they are 2 centimetres wider than the shoulders. The knees face the ceiling and the feet are flexed as if the soles of the feet were against a wall. Lift the arms up to shoulder height with the palms down. **(1)**

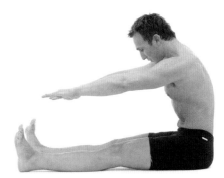

Advanced Transition and Starting Position
From the last Criss-Cross (page 70), roll the head and shoulders back down on to the mat and place the feet on the floor with the knees bent and the inner thighs connected. Place the arms at the sides of the body with the palms down. Breathe in to prepare. Breathe out and roll up through the spine as for Roll-Ups on page 40 or 42. Sit up tall and straighten out the legs. Breathe in, opening the legs so they are 2 centimetres wider than the shoulders and flex the feet. **(1)**

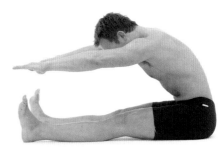

Movement
- The movement is the same as for beginners, except that in this version the arms remain at shoulder height in front of you throughout. **(1 to 3)**

Check Points
The same as for beginners but also:
- Keep the feet flexed and in correct alignment.
- Try and concentrate on keeping the shoulders away from the ears. Imagine being pulled forward from the crown of the head and not by the arms.

Go to Open Leg Rocker on page 76. ➡
Go to Open Leg Rocker on page 78. ➡

Open Leg Rocker

Warning

Not suitable for those with osteoporosis or back problems
caused by nerve damage.

Aim

A more demanding exercise to find your centre which
strengthens the abdominals and stretches the backs
of the legs.

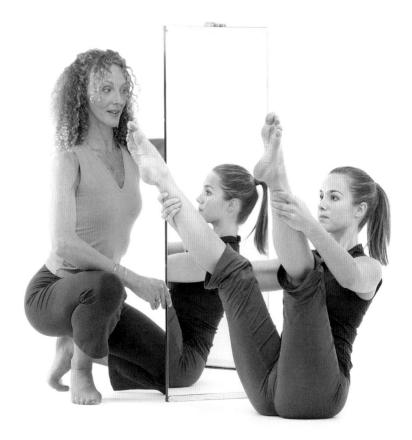

Open Leg Rocker

Transition and Starting Position

From the last Spine Stretch Forward (page 74), bend the knees, opening them as wide as your shoulders. Bring the toes together. Scoop out the lower abdominals. Circle the arms outside the thighs and hold your ankles. If you can't maintain a straight spine while holding your ankles, hold your calves instead. Rock back on to the end of the spine. Find your balance with the toes just off the floor. Lengthen up through the spine, straightening the upper back. **(1)**

Movement

- Breathe in keeping a strong and hollow centre, and slowly straighten the legs into a 'V', keeping the thighs in line with the shoulders. If you have to sacrifice your upright posture in order to have your legs straight, bend your knees a little. Focus straight ahead. **(2)**
- Still breathing in, bring the legs together without letting the shoulders pull forward. Keep the upper back straight. **(3)**
- Breathe out, open the legs back to the 'V' and bend them back to the starting position. Keep the toes just off the floor, maintaining your balance using your navel to spine. **(4)**
- Do 3 to 5 repetitions.

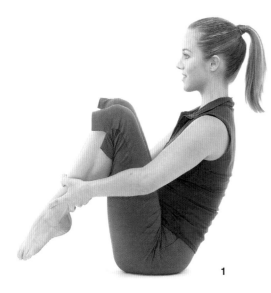

1

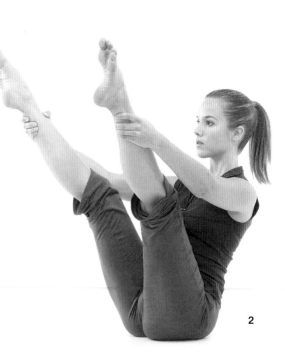

2

Check Points

- Keep the shoulders down the back. Let the hands slide up the legs a little if you have to.
- If you cannot quite straighten the legs without losing a straight back, only extend them as far as you can.
- The trick is to hold the navel to the spine and keep a steady focus.
- Look at your profile in the mirror to check the back is flat.
- Keep the head in line with your shoulders.

Go to Double Leg Circles on page 81.

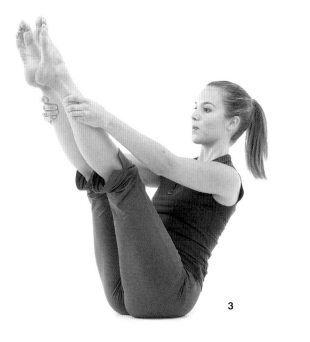

3

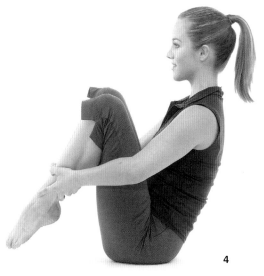

4

Open Leg Rocker

To be attempted only when the intermediate version can be properly accomplished.

Transition and Starting Position

As for the intermediate version. Make sure you balance on the tailbone, toes together and knees shoulder-width apart. Lengthen up through the spine.

Movement

- Breathe out and extend the legs, keeping them shoulder-width apart. They will want to widen. The feet are softly pointed. The arms are straight with the hands holding the ankles firmly. **(1)**
- Breathe in. Start the movement by tucking the sit bones under you and rotating the pelvis. Drop the focus and the chin down and roll back through the spine with control. **(2)**
- Hold the shape. Do not bend the arms or let the legs drop in towards your body. Only roll as far as the shoulders and do not let the head touch the floor. The feet should be just off the floor behind your head. Pause for a milli-second; the arms stay straight; push the legs away. **(3)**
- Breathe out and roll back up through the spine, making sure the lower back rolls through. **(4)**
- Think of the spine as a wheel. As you come back onto the base of the spine, re-stack the upper back and bring the head back up to focus straight ahead of you. Keep navel to spine! This is your brake and the centre of the control of balance. Hold the position for a milli-second. **(5)**
- Do up to 8 rolls backwards and forwards.
- If you cannot hold the position at the roll back or the roll forward, just keep rolling to and fro until you achieve the strength and control to do so.
- To finish, bend the legs back down to the mat, release the ankles and stretch the legs out in front of you, bringing them together.

Check Points

- Your powerhouse is the key.
- Watch that you roll in a straight line.
- Keep the shoulders fixed down the back throughout.
- Do not poke the head forward to pull yourself back up. Keep the eye focus down.
- Feel the work in the abdominals. Check your knees are not turning inwards.
- Roll back with smooth control. You must avoid rolling on to the head and neck. Stop on the shoulders.
- Keep the legs straight.

Go to Double Leg Circles on page 82.

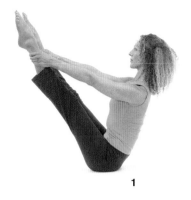

1

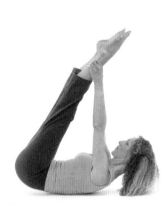

2

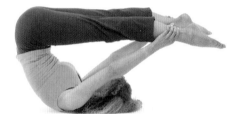

3

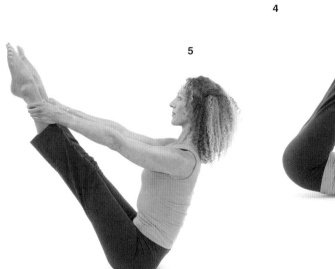

4

5

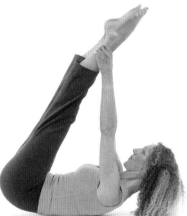

Double Leg Circles

Aim

This is similar to Single Leg Circles (page 49) but
demands more strength in your centre because you have
to keep the pelvis still under the pull of both legs.

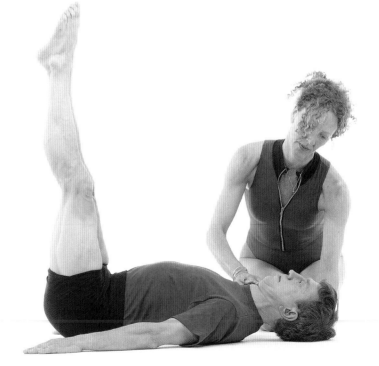

Double Leg Circles

This is also a preparation for the Corkscrew, which has not been included in this book for safety reasons.

Transition and Starting Position

At the end of Open Leg Rocker (page 76), release the legs so they are straight out in front of you. Breathe out and roll down through the spine on to the mat, placing your arms by your sides. Breathe in and, keeping a strong and firm centre, Double Knee Fold (page 28) then straighten the legs, keeping them together, up above the hips. Keep the knees a little bent and connect the inner thighs. The arms are in a low 'V' and the palms are facing down. Anchor yourself through the base of the skull and across the chest and upper back. **(1)**

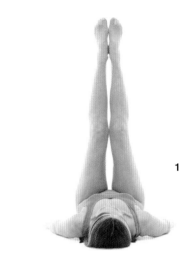

Movement

- Breathe in and move the legs a little to the right. Keep the pelvis still. **(2)**
- Breathe out and circle the legs slightly down towards the floor, then back up to centre. **(3)**
- (Remember the clock face in Single Leg Circles on page 50.) Keep the base of the skull anchored and the ribs pressed into the mat. You will have to use the arms a little to help, but the main worker is the lower abdominal muscle.
- Repeat the circle to the left.
- Keep the circles small and controlled. The back must not arch off the mat and the shoulders must stay square and grounded.
- Do 6 circles, alternating directions.

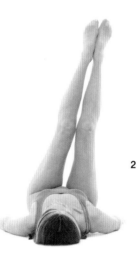

Check Points

- The abdominals must remain scooped into the back.
- Keep the inner thighs connected.
- Keep long through the back of the neck.
- Press the back of the shoulders into the mat without letting the ribs pop up.
- Use breath control to help stabilize the pelvis.

Go to the Saw on page 84. ➡

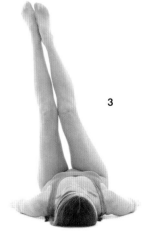

Double Leg Circles

In this version, also called the Baby Corkscrew, the hips twist and the pelvis rotates, mobilizing the lower back. It demands great abdominal strength.

Transition and Starting Position

From the finishing position of the Open Leg Rocker (page 78), where you are seated with the legs straight out in front of you, flex the feet and roll down through the spine. Double Knee Fold (page 28). Straighten the legs completely and point the toes to the ceiling. The legs should be right over the hips. The arms slide out to a low 'V'. Hollow the abdominals, making sure your pelvis and spine are in the neutral position. **(1)**

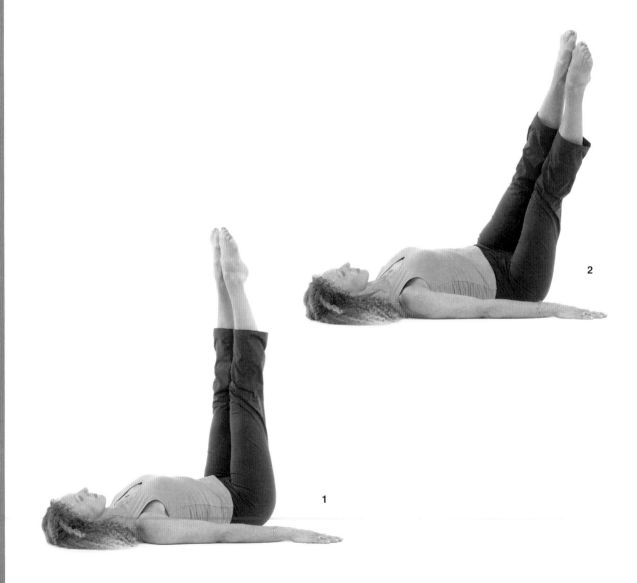

Movement

- Breathe in and take the legs to the right, allowing the left hip to lift slightly from the floor. The legs stay locked together. **(2)**
- Breathe out and lower the legs a little towards the floor, making a circular motion. When the legs are directly back in line with the pelvis, both hip bones should be pressed into the mat, and the pelvis back in neutral. **(3)** Continuing the out breath, circle the legs over to the left allowing the back of the right hip bone to lift slightly from the floor. Keep pressing the spine to the mat. It must not arch. **(4)**
- Repeat the circle to the left.
- Do 6 circles alternating directions.

Check Points

See intermediate version and also:

- Because the legs are straight, you will have to work harder to keep the pelvis from tilting forwards and the back from arching.
- Keep the inner thighs connected.
- Keep the legs straight.
- Do not lower the legs too close to the floor. You must keep the upper back grounded and the abdominals flat and firm. No bulging!

Go to the Saw on page 84.

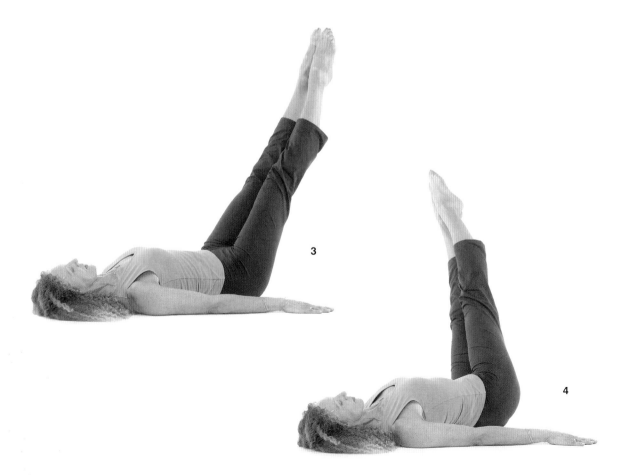

3

4

The Saw

The movement is the same for all levels.

Aim

To work the waistline and empty the lungs of breath. This is a spine stretch, like Spine Stretch Forward (page 73), but with added rotation.

Starting Position (beginners)

Start sitting up with the legs out in front of you and open 2 centimetres wider than the shoulders. Flex the feet. Breathe in and raise the arms up to your sides at shoulder height. The palms are face down. Imagine a pole behind your back and lengthen up, out of the hips. Draw the navel to the spine to prepare. **(1)**

Transition and Starting Position (intermediate)

From the last Double Leg Circle (page 81), bend the knees in towards the chest and lower the feet to the floor in a double leg hinge. Slide the feet slightly away from the buttocks, keeping the inner thighs connected, and then breathe out to roll up slowly through the spine until you are sitting upright. Breathe in and stretch the legs out in front of you along the mat and open them 2 centimetres wider than the shoulders. Flex the feet, and raise the arms up at your sides to shoulder height. The palms are face down. Imagine a pole behind your back and lengthen up, out of the hips. Draw the navel to the spine to prepare. **(1)**

Transition and Starting Position (advanced)

As for the intermediate transition but advanced students roll up with straight legs, the inner thighs connected and the feet flexed. **(1)**

1

The Saw

Movement

- Breathe out and turn the torso, initiating the movement with the head, to your left. The arms move with the shoulder girdle and not independently. Keep exhaling as you stretch the body round and reach your right hand down towards the toes of the left foot. Look down at your knee and lengthen through the back of the neck. Make three small 'sawing' motions on the little toe of the left foot with the little finger of your right hand. Your sit bones must stay anchored to the floor. Rotate the right palm so the thumb faces the floor. Press backwards and upwards to help the twisting of the spine. Wring out every atom of breath. **(2)**
- Breathe in and unravel the stretch, returning to sitting up high out of the hips with a straight spine. Lengthen up the imaginary pole. **(3)**
- Breathe out and repeat the turn to the right.
- Do 6 stretches, alternating directions.
- To finish
  - beginners should lie face down on the mat.
  - intermediates should bend the knees, bring them together, squeeze the inner thighs and roll down through the spine. Place the right arm up by your right ear on the mat and roll over towards it on to your front. If you have a small mat, get into the centre of it.
  - advanced should squeeze the inner thighs together and, keeping the legs straight, roll down through the spine. Place the right arm up by the right ear on the mat and roll over towards it on to your front. Get into the centre of the mat.

Check Points

- The hips remain still and the sit bones anchored. Aim for the little toe but do not lift the opposite sit bone off the mat to achieve this. It doesn't matter if you cannot reach the toes at first.
- Feel the spinal stretch down the spine on the side of your forward arm.
- Keep the shoulders down and away from your ears.
- Keep the feet flexed and the knees straight. They will want to bend a little.
- Feel the lower abdominals sucking in towards the spine and holding the pelvis still.

Go to the Cobra on page 87.

Go to the Swan Dive on page 88.

Go to the Swan Dive on page 89.

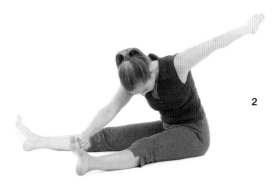

1

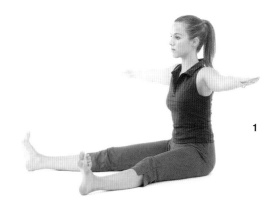

2

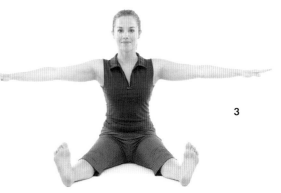

3

The Cobra and the Swan Dive

Aim

To strengthen the spine, the backs of the legs and the buttocks. Now you have warmed up the spine by bending forward you are going to stretch the front of the body and bend the spine backwards.

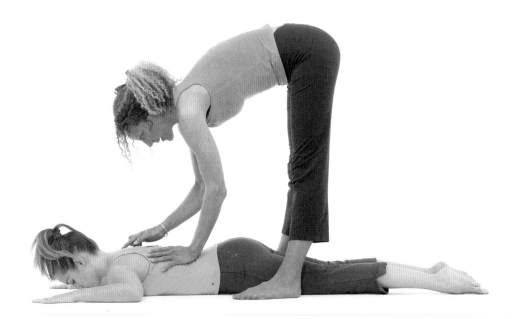

The Cobra

Starting Position for All Levels

Once you are lying on your front, open the legs hip-width apart and turn them out so the knees face out and the front of the hips opens up. Point the feet. Place your hands on either side of your face so the thumbs are about level with your nose. The elbows are bent at right angles. Make sure you are square on the mat. **(1)**

Movement

- Breathe out and draw the navel to the spine, zipping up inside and hollowing the lower abdominals. Imagine you are trying to push a marble away with your nose so your head lifts slightly off the mat and your eye focus falls just ahead of you. Simultaneously, coil the shoulders back and down the spine as you lift them and the chest just off the mat. At this stage you should only be using your back muscles to lift. Once you have come as far as you can using the back, use the arms to help lift the torso off the mat. You might not be able to fully extend the arms. Stop when you have got as far as you can. Keep hollowing the abdominals; they must not sag towards the mat. **(2)**
- Breathe into the ribs, not the tummy, and hold the position.
- Breathe out and slowly lower the torso back to the mat, trying not to use the arms. You will feel the buttocks and backs of the legs working to stabilize the lower body. The face reaches the mat last.
- Breathe in to prepare. Zip up and hollow.
- Breathe out and lift both legs off the mat, keeping them stretched and the upper body calm and relaxed. Do not let the pelvis tilt forward. Keep the pubic bone pressed to the mat and keep the length through the lower back. **(3)**
- Breathe in and lower the legs, reaching away out of the hips.
- Breathe out and repeat the chest lift as above.
- Alternate chest lifts and leg lifts, and do 6 of each.

Check Points

- Keep the shoulders down the back, especially when you are using the arms and during the descent.
- It is imperative to keep a strong firm centre to protect the lower back.
- Think of lengthening out of the waistline and staying long through the lower back.
- Ascend and descend in a straight line.
- Keep long through the back of the neck.
- Keep the legs straight and hold the turn out.

For the final essential exercise, the Seal, go to page 162. ➡

Beginners, go to Single Leg Kicks on page 91. ➡

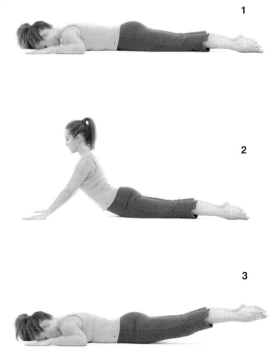

1

2

3

Swan Dive

This exercise strengthens the body and mobilizes the spine like the Cobra (page 87), but uses momentum to aid in increasing spinal flexibility.

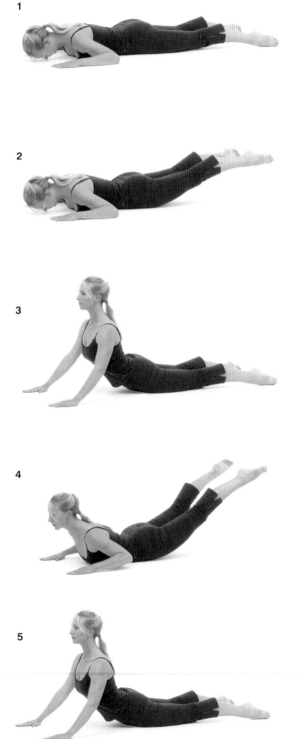

Starting Position (1)
- Get into the same starting position as the Cobra. **(1)**
- Breathe out to prepare, draw the navel to the spine and lift the legs off the mat, stretching through the knees. **(2)**
- Breathe in and peel the head and upper body off the mat using the muscles in your back and then continue to lift the body by pressing into the arms. Keep the back working by trying to keep as little weight as possible on the hands. The legs will lower towards the floor, but keep the muscular tension in the buttocks and the backs of the legs. **(3)**

Movement
- Breathe out and rock forward onto the chest, keeping the head and eye focus up and the hands on the mat. The effort is in the buttocks and backs of the legs. The legs remain straight. Do not let the head drop! Keep the bow shape you made. Watch yourself in the mirror. **(4)**
- Breathe in and lift back up keeping the shoulders down and away from your ears.**(5)**
- Repeat the rocking without hesitating at the top. You should move in a rhythmical rock to and fro.
- Do 6 rocks backwards and forwards.

Check Points
- Use the mirror head on and watch for level legs and correct shoulder stabilization.
- Keep the body in the bow shape. Do not let the head or upper body drop on the rock forward.
- The arms should only help a little.
- Keep the pelvis down on the mat at the height of the rock.
- Breathe!
- Keep navel to spine.

Go to Single Leg Kicks on page 92. ➡

Swan Dive

Starting Position

- Get into the same starting position as for the Intermediate level.
- Breathe out to prepare, zipping up and hollowing and lifting the legs.
- Breathe in and lift the torso to form the bow shape.

Movement

- Breathe out, rock forward and shoot the arms out in front of you in line with your head. **(1)**
- Breathe in and, keeping the arms in line with your head, lift the torso back up. **(2)**
- Breathe out, use the backs of the legs and the buttocks, and rock forward maintaining the shape.
- Do 10 rocks forwards and backwards.

Check Points

As for intermediates but also:

- Keep the arms in line with the head. Do not use them to help with the lift backwards. Imagine holding a big ball.
- Keep the head up and still. It moves with the spine.
- The shoulders are more likely to rise up by your ears. Keep them down the back.

Go to Single Leg Kicks on page 93. ➡

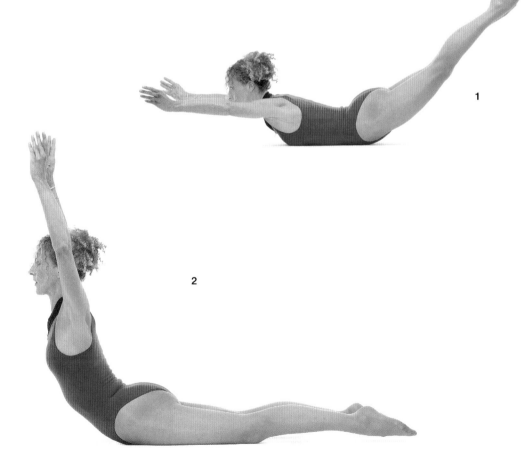

1

2

Single Leg Kicks

Aim

To stretch the front of the body, especially the fronts of the thighs. To tone the buttocks and backs of the legs.

Single Leg Kicks

Starting Position

Lie on your front and fold your hands under your forehead. Connect the inner thighs and point the feet. Draw the shoulders down and lengthen through the back of the neck. Lift the feet just off the mat, keeping the legs straight and engaging the buttocks and the backs of the legs. Keep the top half of your body relaxed.

Movement

- Breathe in and kick the right foot towards the centre of the right buttock, then without lowering the foot, kick in again in a double pulse action – 'in in' not 'in out in'. **(1)**
- Breathe out and repeat the action with the left leg. The legs should pass each other in the air as they change.
- Do 8 kicks with each leg.

Check Points

- Keep the straight leg still and just off the mat as you pulse the bent leg if you can.
- Keep the pubic bone pressed to the mat and the knees lightly resting on it.
- Do not let the pelvis tilt forward, allowing the back to arch. You control the pelvis using the buttocks and the abdominals.
- The pelvis must not rock from side to side.
- Use the mirror to check that the foot comes to the centre of the buttock or turn to look. You will have to put the mirror at your head and lift your head to see.
- Keep the body still; only the legs move.

Go to the Rest Position on page 97.

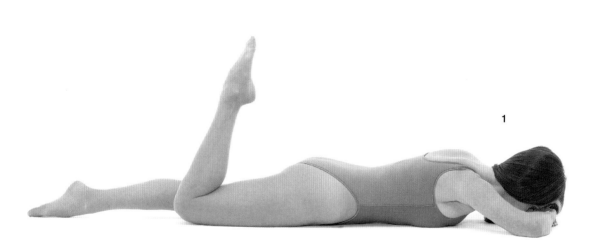

1

Single Leg Kicks

This version includes a stretch right through the front of the body and strengthens the spine and shoulder girdle.

Transition and Starting Position

From the last Swan Dive (page 88), roll the body back onto the mat with your legs together, place your knuckles together just in front of your head and open your elbows, which should be placed a little wider than, and in front of, the shoulders. Press down into the mat with the arms and lift the upper body off it. Keep long through the back of the neck. Push up into the shoulders without causing the back to hump. **(1)**

Movement

- As for beginners but perform the leg kicks while maintaining the position of the upper back. **(2)**
- Do 8 kicks with each leg.

Check Points

As for beginners but also:
- Do not sink into the shoulders or let the head drop.
- Keep the feet lifted off the mat. Try to keep the knees lightly on the mat.
- Do not let the stomach or ribs sink down to the mat. Anchor across the pelvis.

Go to Double Leg Kicks on page 95.

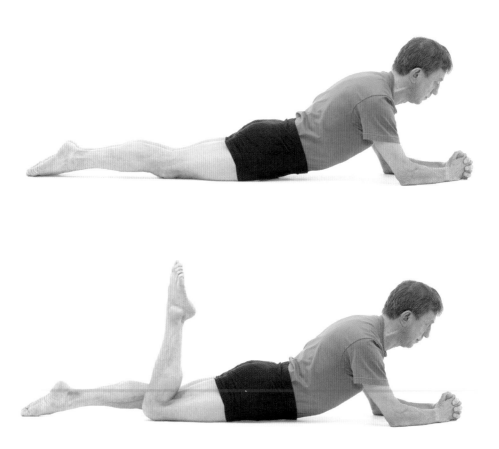

1

2

Single Leg Kicks

This version is harder for the top half of the body because you have to hold your head up and keep the shoulders down which increases the stretch.

Transition and Starting Position

As for intermediate, but place the elbows directly under the shoulders, the hands are in line with the elbows like a sphinx. Make fists with your hands, keeping the thumbs over the fingers. Set the shoulders down the back, press the arms into the mat, push up into the shoulders and then lift your head, tipping it back and focusing on the ceiling. Feel the stretch from your chin to the pubic bone. Keep the mouth closed.

Movement

As for intermediate. **(1)**

Check Points

As for intermediate but also:

- Keep the pressure of the arms into the mat.
- Keep your mouth closed.
- Really concentrate on keeping the collarbones away from the ears.

Go to Double Leg Kicks on page 96. ▬▶

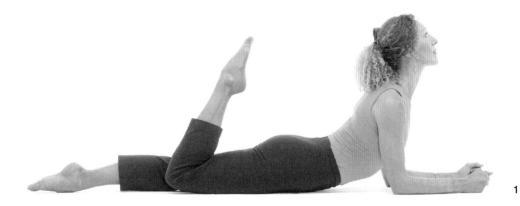

1

Double Leg Kicks

Aim

To open the shoulders and chest, to tone the buttocks and
the backs of the thighs and to strengthen the spine.

Double Leg Kicks

Transition and Starting Position

From the last Single Leg Kick (page 92), roll down onto the mat, placing your right cheek on it. Circle the arms down and round until the hands meet over your back. Clasp the right fingers with the left hand and place them as far up the back as possible. Press the elbows to the floor or as close to the floor as possible. (You might need to lower the hands down the back a little to find a comfortable position.) The shoulders remain down the back. Your legs remain connected in parallel, with the feet just off the mat. **(1)**

Movement

- Breathe out to prepare, drawing the navel to the spine and anchoring across the pelvis using the buttock muscles to help.
- Breathe in to kick both feet towards the buttocks keeping the legs together. Do a triple pulse – 'in in in'. **(2)**
- Breathe out and open the legs slightly as you straighten them away from the buttocks. Lift them as high as possible off the mat while keeping the knees straight. Simultaneously, lift the head and chest, keeping a long neck. Release your hands and straighten the arms down the body, pressing them slightly up towards the ceiling with the palms facing inwards. Reach up and away. Open the chest and keep the abdominals scooped. **(3)**
- Breathe in and bend the legs so the feet come back towards the buttocks, keeping the legs together. Repeat the beats, with the hands rejoined behind the back and the pelvis still anchored to the mat. Place the left cheek down on the mat this time.
- Breathe out and release into the back and leg lift.
- Repeat up to 6 times.

Check Points

- Keep the pelvis anchored.
- Try not to pinch the shoulder blades but roll the shoulders backwards.
- Lengthen through the back of the neck.
- Keep the legs straight as you lift them up behind you.
- Place the elbows back as close to the floor as possible during the beats.
- Alternate the cheeks.

Go to the Rest Position on page 97.

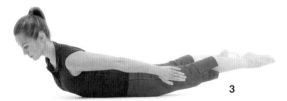

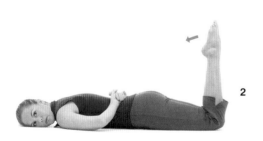

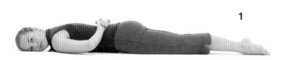

Double Leg Kicks

Much harder as the legs remain connected along with the hands.

Transition and Starting Position
As for intermediate. **(1)**

Movement
- As for intermediate, but breathe out and beat the legs **(2)** and breathe in as you straighten the legs, keeping them together and off the floor. Pull the clasped hands down past your bottom. The palms will turn in to face up to your head. Lift the chin to the ceiling. Feel the front of the shoulders stretching as you pull the hands away. Keep the abdominals lifting up into the back. **(3)**
- Breathe out to lower down, placing the left cheek on the mat and bending the arms back to repeat the kicks.
- Do up to 8 repetitions.

Check Points
As for intermediate version but also:
- Keep the inner thighs connected.
- As you stretch the arms away, ease the shoulders down the back.
- Keep the shoulders down as you bend the elbows back as close to the floor as possible, and place the clasped hands high up the back.
- Keep the mouth closed as you lift the chin.
- You may reverse the breathing if you cannot hold navel to spine during the lift.

Go to the Rest Position on page 97. ➡

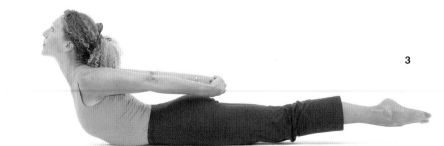

1

2

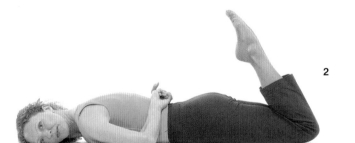

3

Rest Position

Aim
To stretch and relax the spine after the back extensions.

Starting Position
From the last Single Leg Kick (page 91) or Double Leg Kick (page 95 or 96), place the hands beneath the shoulders, stabilize them, brace the stomach and extend the arms to lift the torso off the floor. The knees are bent and open a little, the toes are together. Push the sit bones back on to the heels. Leave the arms stretched out, shoulder-width apart, and soften the elbows. Relax the head down and release the lower back. Take 6 deep breaths.

Check Points
- If you feel uncomfortable in the neck and shoulders, bring the arms closer to you.
- Release all round the buttocks and groin.
- Stretch the ribs with each in breath.
- Check you are sitting on both sit bones equally by looking between the legs.

Go to Side Kicks on page 121. ⇒
Go to the Neck Pull on page 99. ⇒
Go to the Neck Pull on page 100. ⇒

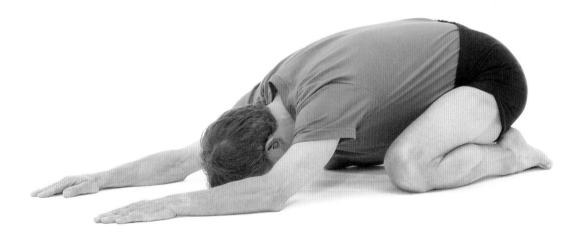

Neck Pull

Aim

To stretch the spine, including the neck. To strengthen the trunk flexors muscles.

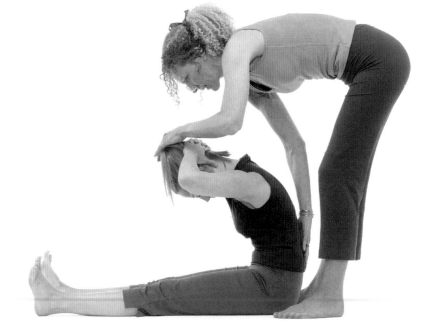

Neck Pull

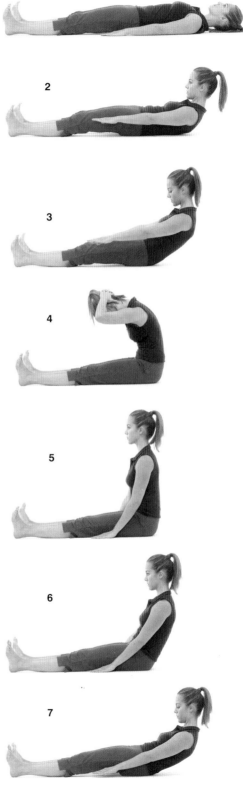

Transition and Starting Position

From the Rest Position (page 97), lengthen the body back out over the mat, supporting the trunk with the arms. The knees should still be on the mat and the body flat, like a plank. Lower the torso to the mat. Straighten the legs and place the left arm alongside your left ear. Roll over towards the arm to lie on your back. If you have a small mat, get into the centre again. Put the arms down beside the hips with the palms down. Open the legs to hip-width apart and flex the feet. Draw the navel to the spine. Make sure you are straight and the pelvis and spine are in neutral. **(1)**

Movement

- Breathe in, nod the chin down and, lifting the head, slowly roll the spine off the mat. Coil right into your centre, like a caterpillar rolling into a ball. **(2 and 3)**
- Breathe out as you curl the head and body into the navel and place the hands over the back of the skull with the elbows open. Rest the hands on the skull and release the head and jaw. You should feel a gentle stretch from the tailbone to the skull. **(4)**
- Breathe in and roll up through the spine until the shoulders are directly over the hips. Place your arms back alongside your body. **(5)**
- Breathe out, squeeze the buttocks and hollow navel to spine to initiate a smooth roll back through the spine down to the mat. Keep the spine long as you roll through it. Focus slightly down and check the hips stay square. **(6, 7 and 1)**
- Do up to 5 repetitions.

Check Points

- The roll up and down must be smooth, working through the lower back. Do not hinge up from the hips.
- Keep the arms sliding along the mat as you roll up, keeping the shoulders down and the chest open.
- As you roll up, slide the ribs towards the hips and then press down in the waistline to roll through it.
- Keep the abdominals scooped in. No bulging. Push through the heels and down through the back of the legs.

Go to Spine Twists on page 112. ➡

Neck Pull

Tougher on the abdominals with the extra
weight of the arms. Requires great strength
and flexibility of the spine.

Transition and Starting Position
As for intermediate but, instead of placing the arms down
by the body, you circle them up and clasp the hands
behind the back of the skull. Open the elbows down to the
floor if possible, without letting the shoulders rise. **(1)**

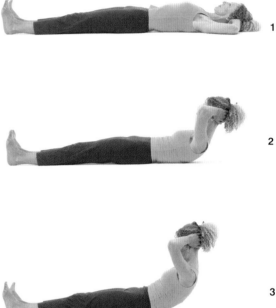

1

Movement
- As for the intermediate version.
- Your hands are already behind your skull for the neck
  pull. Keep the elbows open throughout the exercise.
- Do up to 5 repetitions. **(2 to 9)**

2

Check Points
- You must be able to roll smoothly through the spine
  with the arms in this position. Do not allow the elbows
  to close in towards each other.
- Use the energy going through the heels to help ground
  the legs to the mat.
- Keep the head at the end of the spine as you roll down.
  You coil up but remain lengthened to roll down.
- Initiate the roll-down by squeezing the buttocks and
  pinning the navel to the spine.

3

Go to the Scissors on page 104.

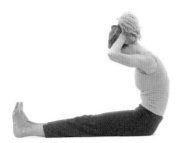

4

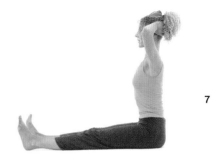

7

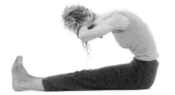

5

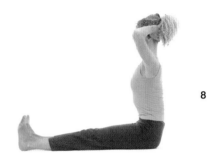

8

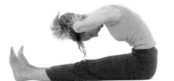

6

9

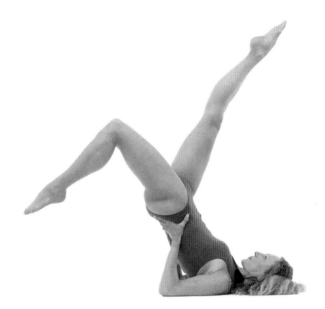

The following three exercises, Scissors, Bicycle/Reverse Bicycle and Shoulder Bridge are all performed on the shoulders and are only for students at an advanced level. Without the correct technique these exercises are firstly, dangerous and secondly, ineffective. All the shoulder stand exercises encourage blood circulation to the brain and counteract the normal forces of gravity which tend to compress the spine.

Scissors

Aim

To stretch the front of the hips, work the backs of the legs, the buttocks and the abdominals which help maintain the position.

Transition and Starting Position

From the last Neck Pull (page 100), place the arms in a low 'V' at your sides, palms down. Anchor yourself through the back of the skull, across the chest and down the back of the arms. Bring the legs together, softly point the feet and bend the knees. Stabilize the pelvis, hollow the abdominals and lift the feet off the ground. Straighten the legs above the hips. Breathe in and bring the legs slightly over your torso. Breathe out and roll the spine up off the mat pushing the toes towards the ceiling as for Jack Knife (page 116) and Roll Over (page 46). Find your balance in the shoulder stand. **(1)** You must not press into the skull; the head must rest on the floor and not aid in balancing you. Breathe in and carefully lift the forearms off the mat and place the hands on the back of the pelvis so the backs of the hips are resting on the heels of your hands. The hands only help to support the stand; it is your abdominals and the buttocks which maintain it.

1

Movement

- Breathe out and then in, stretch the toes up towards the ceiling and lift out of the hips.
- Breathe out and push the left leg away from you, towards the wall in front of you and down towards the floor. Simultaneously, bring the right leg towards you. Do not allow it to drop right down, you are trying to make an even split. The pelvis stays still with the hips square. Use your hands to check for unwanted movement. **(2)**
- Breathe in and change legs, moving them so they 'scissor' past each other over the hips.
- Breathe out to stretch the right leg away towards the wall in front of you and down towards the floor.
- Do up to 10 changes.

Check Points

- Do not lose the work in the abdominals and buttocks and end up resting on your hands and elbows only.
- Use the mirror in profile to check your even split. Only check it briefly because turning the head in this position should not be sustained.
- Keep the body weight on the shoulders and upper back and *not* the neck.
- Keep the legs straight; the leg reaching away will want to bend.
- Keep the knees facing straight ahead and in line with the hip sockets.
- Feel the front of the hips stretching as you reach the leg forward, away from your face. Use the back of the leg to draw the leg away.
- If your wrists hurt, try putting less weight on them or change the angle of the wrist with the lower arm.

Continue with the Bicycle/Reverse Bicycle on page 106. ➡

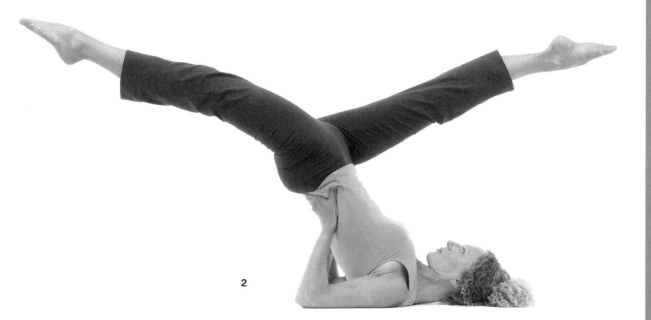

2

The Bicycle / Reverse Bicycle

Aim

To stretch the muscles in the front of the hip and the leg.
To tone the backs of the legs.

Starting Position

Remaining in the shoulder stand from the Scissors (page 104), bring both legs together and check your position: pelvis square; navel to spine. Reach the toes up and out of the hips. **(1)**

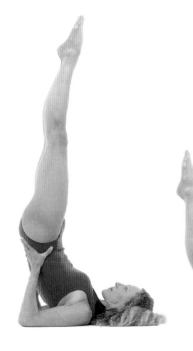

2

3

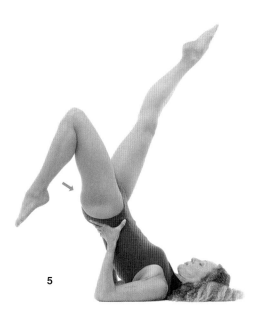

Movement

- Breathe in and stretch the left leg away down towards the floor and the wall in front of you. Allow the right leg to move a few centimetres towards your face. A *few* centimetres! **(2 and 3)**
- When you can reach no further with the left leg, bend the left knee in, trying to touch your buttock with your left foot, then straighten it back up over the hip, in a bicycling motion. Keep the foot, knee and hip in one line. **(4 and 5)**
- Breathe out as you straighten the left leg back up and start cycling the right leg out and away. The left leg moves slightly towards your face. The pelvis remains stable. Look at the pictures carefully, paying particular attention to the positions of the legs during each part of the cycling motion.
- Cycle 6 times one way, then reverse the cycling and do 6 the other way.

The Bicycle / Reverse Bicycle

Reverse Bicycle

- Bring the legs together after the last bicycle.
- Breathe out and bend the left knee, trying to keep the knees together and fixed in space. Reach the toes of your left foot down towards your right buttock then stretch it out and bring it back up to above the hip. **(1a to 5a)**
- Breathe in as you finish bringing the left leg up and start bending the right leg, trying not to displace the right knee in space. Do not let it drop down to your face. Continue to reach the toes to the buttock and then stretch the leg in a reversed cycling motion, as if pedalling backwards.
- Do 6 repetitions in all.

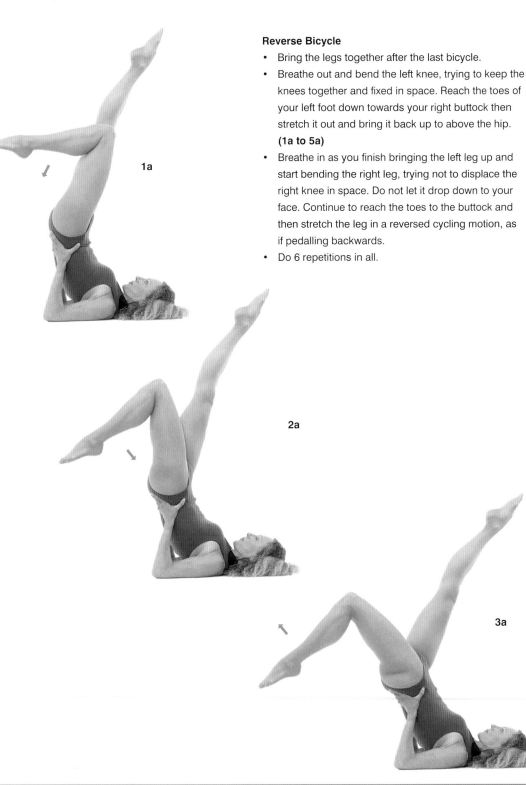

1a

2a

3a

Check Points

- Feel a stretch down the front of the thighs and over the front of the hips.
- Use the buttocks and the backs of the legs.
- Keep the legs moving in one plane. The legs might get pulled out to the side, out of line with the hip socket. Watch them.
- Keep the trunk and pelvis still.
- Pin the navel to the spine and keep a firm centre.
- Keep the weight off the head and on the shoulders. Keep the shoulders away from the ears.
- Breathe!

Go to the Shoulder Bridge on page 110. ➡

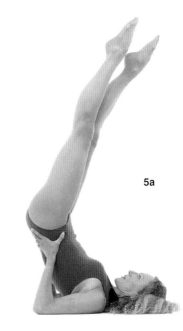

5a

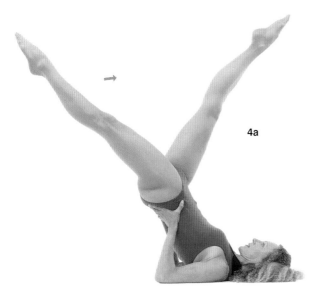

4a

Shoulder Bridge

Aim

This is a dynamic exercise and requires real work from the supporting leg and hip. It requires a flexible lower back.

Transition and Starting Position

If you can manage it, this is a great transition and a favourite of mine.

Bring the legs back together after the last Reverse Bicycle (page 107) and stay in a shoulder stand. Adjust the hands so the fingers wrap round the front of the hip bones and the heels of your hands support the back of the pelvis. You may need to lower your shoulder stand slightly by moving your elbows outwards. Stretch the right leg out and away and keep the left leg reaching up to the ceiling. As the right leg lowers towards the floor, allow the pelvis to rotate, bend the right knee and place the right foot firmly on the floor with the toes pointing straight forwards. The left leg ends up straight above the left hip and is still stretching towards the ceiling. Soften down the ribcage and adjust the hand if your back is over-arched. The right buttock and muscles at the back of the leg should work hard to keep the pelvis square. There should not be a lot of weight on your elbows; use the supporting leg to bear the weight. Check your body is square and the ribs are level and your right foot and leg are aligned with the hip. **(1)**

1

Movement

- Breathe out to prepare. Navel to spine.
- Breathe in and flex the left foot. Lower the left leg towards the floor in line with the hip. Lengthen over that hip keeping the pelvis still. It will want to tilt forward. Press through the heel and feel the backs of the legs and the buttocks working, supporting from underneath. **(2)**
- Breathe out and sweep the leg straight back up, pointing the toes.
- Slowly lower the leg and quickly raise it 3 times, then breathe in and bend the left knee in. Breathe out and place the left foot on the floor. The foot is under the knee and toes and facing straight forward.
- Breathe in and bend the right knee up over the hip.
- Breathe out and straighten the right leg up.
- Repeat the lowers and lifts 3 times and then change legs again.
- Work up to 3 sets of 3 kicks on each leg, alternating legs.
- To finish, place your arms by your sides on the mat and curl the spine back on to the floor, one vertebra at a time.

Check Points

- Keep the body and pelvis square.
- Feel the foot firmly on the floor as it supports the rest of the body.
- Keep the pressure off the elbows!
- Kick the leg in alignment with the hip.
- Do not allow the torso or pelvis to twist.
- Do not forget the upper body. Lengthen through the crown of the head and keep the shoulders down.
- Do not flare the ribcage.
- Check your leg positioning in the mirror. The foot should be under the knee.

Go to Spine Twists on page 112.

2

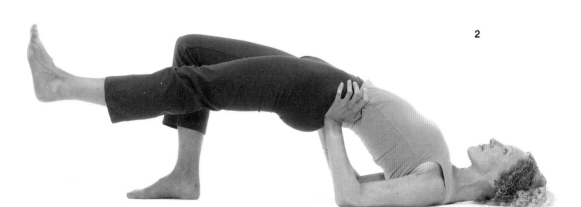

Spine Twists

Aim
To work the waistline and rotate the spine.

Transition and Starting Position (intermediate)
From the last Neck Pull (page 99), roll up once more through the spine. Once the shoulders are over the hips, sit up with a straight back and close the legs together. The feet are flexed. Squeeze the inner thighs together and squeeze the buttocks, lifting up out of the hips. Open your arms and bring them to the sides at shoulder height. You should be able to see your hands in your peripheral vision.

Transition and Starting Position (advanced)
From the finishing position of the Shoulder Bridge (page 110), straighten out the legs and close them together, squeeze the inner thighs and flex the feet. The arms are alongside the body. Roll up through the spine and re-stack the vertebrae so you are sitting up with a straight back. Keep the feet flexed. Squeeze the buttocks and open the arms out to your sides at shoulder height, palms facing down. Sit up out of the hips. **(1)**

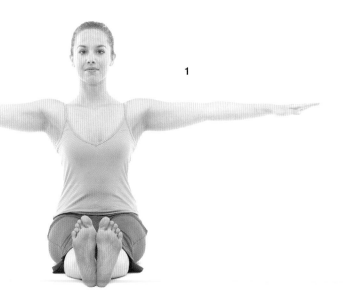

1

Spine Twists

Movement

- Breathe in and lengthen the spine up an imaginary pole. **(1)**
- Breathe out and, initiating the movement with the head, turn to the right, turning the ribs round a stable pelvis. Keep squeezing the inner thighs. There is no movement in the hips, legs or feet. Imagine you have a pole across your arms, so you do not move them independently. They move with the shoulder girdle. **(2)**
- At the very end of the twist, breathe out every atom of air, like wringing out a wet towel, and push the chest round a little bit more. **(3)**
- Breathe in and rotate the chest back to the centre. Sit up!
- Breathe out and repeat to the left. Make sure you turn round the central axis of your spine. It is common to pull off to one side. Use the mirror face on. Feel the sit bones anchored equally to the mat.
- Do 6 twists alternating directions.

Check Points

- Look at your hand as you turn.
- Keep the navel to spine.
- Keep the feet flexed.
- There is no movement in the pelvis.
- If you cannot sit up with a straight back, sit on a telephone directory.
- Keep the head aligned with the spine and the tip of the ear in line with the shoulder.
- Keep the arms fixed in a line with the shoulders.
- Keep the shoulders down.
- You should check your posture from the side using the mirror in profile as well as in front of you.

Go to Jack Knife on page 115.
Go to Jack Knife on page 116.

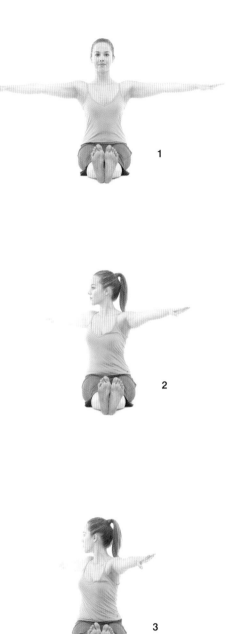

1

2

3

Jack Knife

Aim

To strengthen the abdominals and lengthen the spine
in inversion using gravity.

Jack Knife

Transition and Starting Position

From the last Spine Twist (page 113), bring both arms forward, shoulder-width apart and level with the shoulders. Bend the knees slightly, and roll down through the spine. Place your arms in a low 'V' on the mat, with the palms down. Bend the knees in and, making sure to hollow the abdominals, hinge the legs up over the body and stretch them to the ceiling. **(1)**

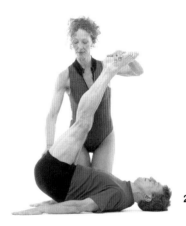

1

Movement

- Breathe in and hinge the legs over the body to an angle of approximately 45 degrees, keeping the legs straight.
- Breathe out and use the lower abdominals to lift the hips off the mat. **(2)**
- Once the lower back is lifted, push the toes straight up to the ceiling in a jack-knife motion.
- You will feel the work move from the abdominals to the buttocks and backs of the legs. **(3)**
- You are balanced on your shoulders and not on the head and neck!
- Breathe in and reach up out of the hips, toes stretching to the ceiling. **(4)**
- Breathe out and, with great control, bring the legs back towards the body, no more than 45 degrees, and roll the spine and hips back to the mat. This takes great abdominal strength. You will feel the backs of the arms working. Keep the back of the neck long, chin down and the shoulders pressing into the mat. Keep reaching the arms away past the hips. Bring the legs back to the starting position, over the hips and finish your exhalation.
- Breathe in and start again.
- Do up to 5 repetitions.

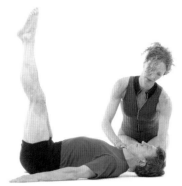

2

Check Points

See page 116.

Go to Side Kicks on page 121. ➡

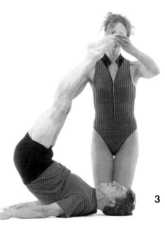

3

4

Jack Knife

Transition and Starting Position
As for intermediate, but roll down through the spine with straight legs and flexed feet.

Movement
- This is very hard to perform correctly and takes a great deal of practice.
- If you become competent with the intermediate version you can increase the difficulty by keeping the feet further away from you as you push up on to the shoulders into a high shoulder stand and then try to roll down with the feet over the hips. **(1)**
- The work moves from the lower abdominals to the upper abdominals **(2)** and then to the buttocks and the backs of the legs as you reach the feet to the ceiling when jack-knifing up. **(3)**
- Keep the legs facing straight towards you and the inner thighs connected, especially on the way down. **(4)**
- The shoulders will lift off the mat and the head will tip back or come up off the floor if you do not work to keep them down.
- Do not lose the abdominal contraction and keep your centre flat and firm. The descent is controlled by the abdominals.

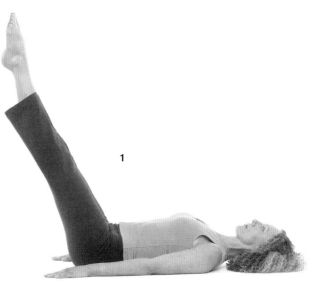

1

Check Points
- The work moves from the lower abdominals to the upper abdominals and then to the buttocks and the backs of the legs as you reach the feet to the ceiling when jack knifing up.
- Keep the legs facing straight towards you and the inner thighs connected, especially on the way down.
- The shoulders will lift off the mat and the head will tip back or come up off the floor if you do not work to keep them down.
- Do not lose the abdominal contraction and keep your centre flat and firm. The descent is controlled by the abdominals.

Go to Side Kicks on page 121. ➡

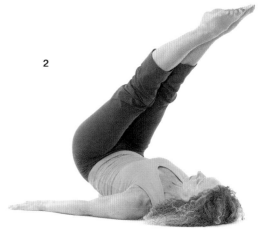

2

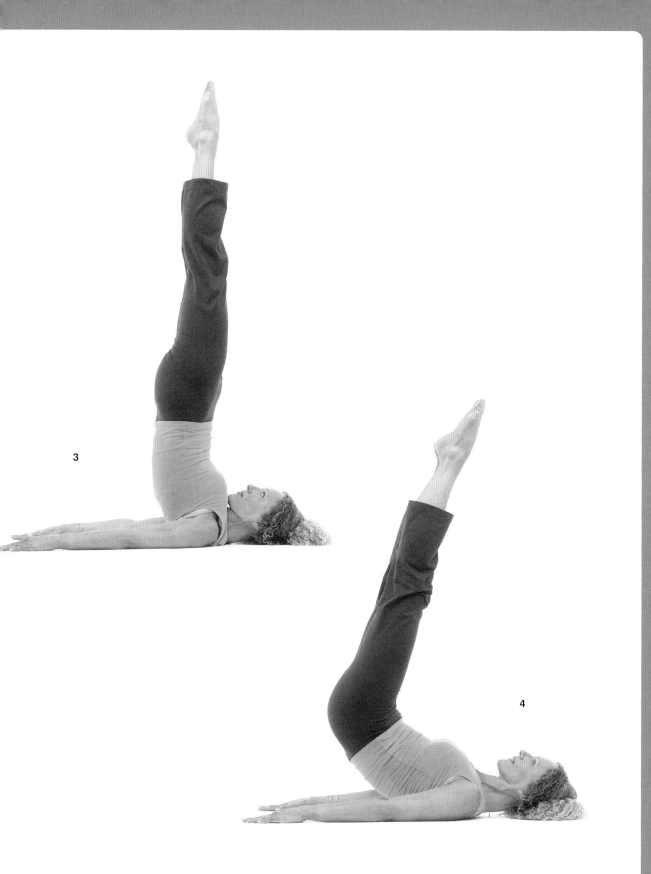

3

4

Side-lying Series

Side Kicks

Aim

To work the hips, while maintaining good core stability.
To stretch the front of the hips and the backs of the legs.

The movement is the same for all levels; only the
transitions and starting positions are different. Stay on the
same side and do the following 2 exercises, then turn on
the other side and repeat all 3.

Transition and Starting Position (beginners)

From the Rest Position (page 97), roll up through the spine
until you are on your knees and sitting back on your heels.
Use the arms to help if necessary. Lie on your left side,
towards the edge of the mat in a straight line, shoulder
over shoulder, hip over hip and ankle over ankle. Breathe
in to prepare, and zip up and hollow. Breathe out and lift
both legs so they are just off the mat. Bring them forward,
from the tops of the legs, so they are at approximately 45
degrees to the body. Lower them back down to the floor.
Place your right hand on the floor in front of your chest,
with the elbow bent. Prop your head up on your left hand
with the left elbow in line with the shoulders and hips. Lift
the right leg up a few inches so it is level with your hip. The
knee points straight forward. Keeping the pelvis still, ease
the leg backwards so it is extended just behind the hip.
Do not let the back arch. **(1)**

Transition and Starting Position (intermediate)

From the last Jack Knife (page 115), bend the legs and
place the feet on the mat. Extend the legs and roll onto the
left side. Assume the starting position described for
beginners. **(1)**

Transition and Starting Position (advanced)

As for intermediate transition. The starting position is
almost the same, but you remove the right hand from the
floor and place it over the right ear and open the elbow.
There should be a straight line from elbow to elbow which
must be maintained throughout. The tendency is for the
upper elbow and shoulder to drop backwards.

Side Kicks

Movement

- Breathe in and, with control, sweep the right leg forward, hinging from the hip. The pelvis and back must not move. As you reach the end of the sweep forward, draw the leg slightly back, flex the foot, then pulse it a little further forward. **(2)**
- This adds an extra stretch to the back of the leg and demands control of the movement. Keep the upper body completely still!
- Breathe out, point the foot and sweep the leg back, trying to get the straight knee just behind the hip bone. Use the top of the back of the leg and the buttock to make the movement, and think of pressing the hip forward to counteract the pull. The upper body remains fixed. Use the mirror face on. **(3)**
- Do up to 10 sweeps forwards and backwards.

Check Points

- Only the leg moves.
- Focus straight ahead.
- The pelvis and spine do not move.
- Do not collapse on to the supporting arm under your head. The armpit should be off the mat with the ribcage resting on the mat.
- Do not grip in the muscles down the front of the thigh. The work is in the haunches.
- The extra kick is a pulse forward and requires effort and control.
- Keep the neck long and the shoulders down, away from your ears.
- Lengthen through the crown of the head.

Stay lying on the left side for Side Kick Lift on page 122.

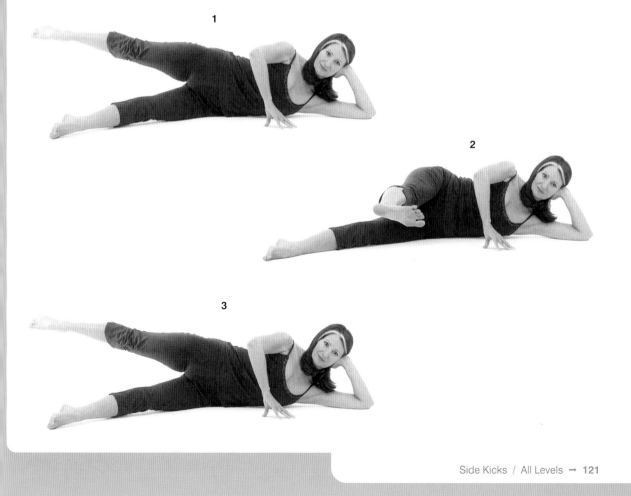

Side Kick Lift

Aim
To tone the legs and mobilize and strengthen the hips.

Starting Position
From the last Side Kick (page 121), lower the right leg back on top of the left leg. Rotate the leg from the hip, so the knee faces up to the ceiling. This is a small movement and the knee might not face directly up. Turn it as far as you can without disturbing the pelvis. **(1)**

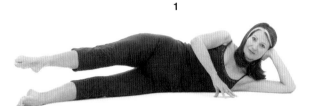

Movement
- Breathe in and kick the right leg straight up. Do not let the underneath waistline drop to the mat. Think of lifting the leg long out of the hip. **(2)**
- Breathe out and flex the foot at the height of the kick, then slowly lower the leg back down to meet the left leg. Keep the turn-out and keep the foot flexed. **(3)** Imagine you are pushing it back down against a strong up-draught.
- Do up to 10 repetitions.

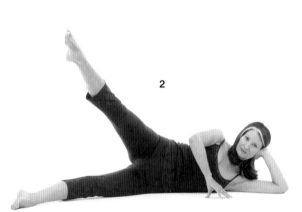

Check Points
- Reach right out of the hip as you kick the leg. Do not let the hip hike up towards the lower ribs.
- Keep the whole spine long from the crown of the head to the toes.
- Keep lifted in the upper body. Have a glance or two at the leg and foot to check placement and turn-out, but otherwise look straight ahead.
- Keep the pelvis facing straight forward, it will want to roll backwards.
- Keep the pelvis and spine in neutral. When turning out, be careful not to tuck the tailbone under.

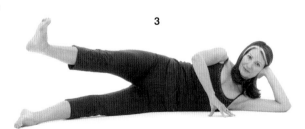

Go to Small Circles Side-lying on page 123.

➡ ➡ ➡

Small Circles Side-lying

Aim

To work the high buttock muscles, the haunches and trunk and pelvic stablilizers.

Starting Position

Check your alignment.

Movement

- Breathe in to prepare, hollowing the abdominals.
- Breathe out and lift the right leg just off the left leg with the toes softly pointed. Do not lock the knee. Try and keep it soft but not bent! **(1)**
- Breathe in and start circling the leg forward and up.
- Breathe out and continue to circle the leg back, bringing it just behind the left leg to brush the left heel. The circle is no bigger than the circumference of a football.
- Do 8 to 10 circles forward and then reverse the circle.

Check Points

- The pelvis must not move. Keep hollowing navel to spine.
- Lengthen out of the hip joint. Use the hollowing of the lower abdominals to keep the movement only in the leg.
- Do not slouch in the upper body. Think length.
- Keep the foot in good alignment with the knee and the hip.
- Circle from the hip.
- You should feel the work in the back of the hips and in the haunches.

All levels roll over on to your right side and assume the appropriate starting position for Side Kicks. Repeat the Side Kicks, the Side Kick Lift and the Small Circles Side-lying with the right leg. Advanced students, do not forget, you do not use the right hand to help support you for the first exercise.

Roll on to your front.

Go to Heel Beats on page 124.

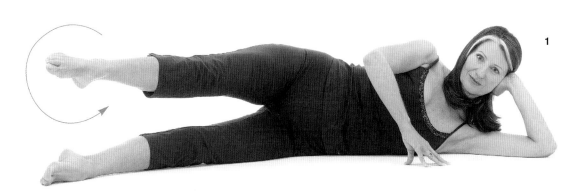

1

Heel Beats

Aim
To help open up the front of the hips after the Side-lying Leg Series.

Starting Position
At the end of Small Circles Side-lying (page 123) roll on to your front. Close the legs together and, rotating from the hip, turn out the legs so the knees face out to the sides. Fold the hands under the forehead.

Movement
- Breathe in to prepare.
- Breathe out and lift both legs about 2 centimetres off the mat. Keep the knees straight and hold the turn-out. **(1)**
- Breathe in and beat the heels together rapidly 5 times. **(2)**
- Breathe out and continue beating the heels for another 5 beats.
- Do 30 beats in all.
- To finish, roll on to your left side.

Check Points
- Keep the legs straight and hold the turn-out.
- Keep the abdominals hollowed and the pubic bone pressed into the mat.
- Try to relax the upper body.

Go to the Torpedo on page 126. ➡
Go to the Torpedo on page 128. ➡
Go to the Torpedo on page 129. ➡

1

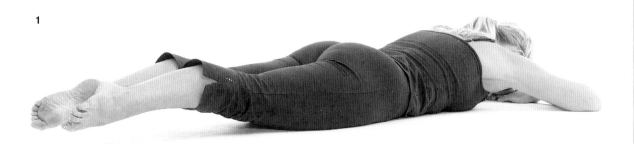

2

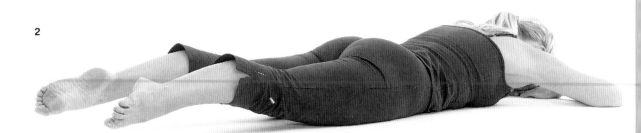

Torpedo

There are many exercises described within the Pilates technique as Side Lifts. The Torpedo is the most effective and works all the required muscles in one exercise.

Aim
To slim the hips and legs and trim the waistline.
To learn balance.

Torpedo

Starting Position

Lie on your left side in a straight line. Use the edge of the mat as a guideline to see where you are. You should have hip over hip, shoulder over shoulder and foot over foot. Your left arm is in a straight line above your head and you rest your head on the arm. Place your right arm on the mat or floor in front of your chest with the elbow bent like a stand. The toes are softly pointed. **(1)**

Movement

- Breathe out to prepare, tightening your buttocks and hollowing your lower abdominals. Connect the inner thighs.
- Breathe in and lift both legs together straight off the mat as high as you can without disturbing the pelvis. Keep the navel to the spine. **(2)**
- Breathe out and lift the right leg up above the left, keeping the knees facing straight forward. Do not allow the back to arch. Keep the right leg raised off the mat. **(3)**
- Breathe in and bring the legs back together, so the inner thighs meet. **(4)**
- Breathe out and bring the legs down to the mat, resisting a little with the right leg so you can feel the inner thighs working. **(5)**
- Do up to 10 repetitions, turn onto your right side and repeat.

Check Points

- Stay long and lifted through the waistline.
- Keep the abdominals scooped in, especially during the initial lift.
- Do not put a lot of pressure on the supporting hand. It is only there to help maintain balance. Try using one finger.
- Be careful the legs do not move forwards or backwards from the hip line during the exercise.
- Do not allow the pelvis to roll backwards, especially when lifting the top leg away from the bottom.
- Try and keep the buttocks working. They will also help maintain the balance.
- When the legs are together, keep the ankles together (unless you are knock-kneed, in which case, keep the knees together).
- Your energy should be moving out through the crown of the head and away through the feet.

Go to the Teaser on page 131.

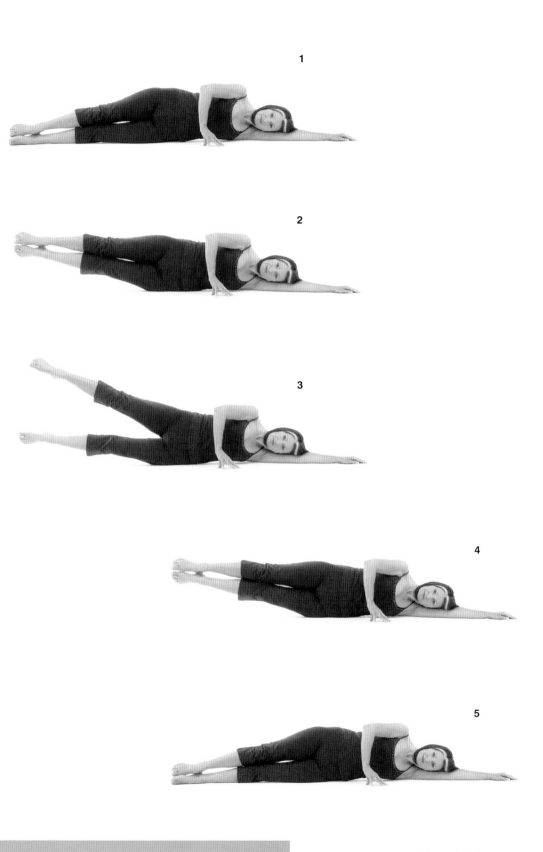

Torpedo

Transition and Starting Position

At the end of Heel Beats (page 124) roll onto your left side and lie in a straight line as for beginners. However, this time you do not have a supporting hand on the floor. When lying on the left side, the right arm rests on the right side of the body and vice versa. **(1)**

Movement

As for beginners. **(2)** If you can't balance you can also raise the head just off the arm. To stop your shoulder rolling forward place your palm on your buttock instead of your thigh. Keep the ribs softly closed.

Check Points

As for beginners.

Go to the Teaser on page 132. ➡

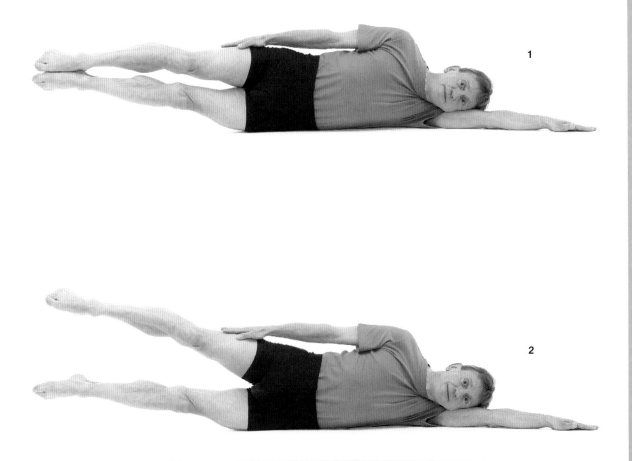

1

2

Torpedo

Transition and Starting Position

The transition is the same as for intermediate but the starting position is another step to finding your core strength and your balance. Lie on the left side with both arms placed in an oval above your head. **(1)** The left elbow should be just off the mat so you do not use it to help you balance. You have to lift the head and torso slightly. **(2)**

Movement

As for the intermediate version. **(3 to 5)**

Check Points

As for beginners but also:

- Do not lift the head out of alignment with the spine.
- Try to keep the elbow off the floor.
- The more you stretch out long and thin the better you will maintain your balance.
- Keep the movements small and neat at first. Once you are stable make them a little bigger.

Go to the Teaser on page 134. ➡

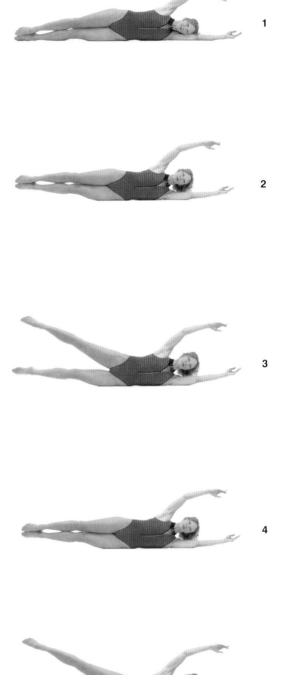

1

2

3

4

5

Teaser

Aim

A very demanding exercise which strengthens the legs,
thighs and abdominals and helps you find your centre.

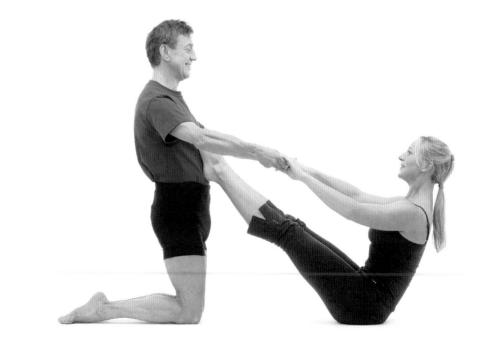

Teaser

Starting Position

Place the mat so the end of it is against a wall. Lie on the mat and bend the knees in towards the body and then rest your feet, with your legs at about a 45-degree angle from the body, against the wall, with the inner thighs connected. Place your arms alongside the body with the palms down. A friend can support you. **(1)**

Movement

- Breathe in to prepare. Zip up and hollow the lower abdominals.
- Breathe out and drop the chin down to begin a smooth roll-up through the spine. Raise your arms at the same time, with fingers reaching to your toes so the arms are parallel with the legs. Make sure you roll through the lower back and do not hinge up from the hips.
- Breathe in and hold the position, keeping the navel to spine.
- Breathe out and roll back down through the spine, placing the arms back by your sides.
- Do up to 6 repetitions.
- If you cannot roll up to form the 'V' shape, just roll as far as you can, hold the position and then roll back.

Check Points

- Peel each vertebra off the mat.
- Coil the shoulders down the back.
- Do not poke the head forward.
- Sit up to a high 'V' keeping the chest open.
- Keep the inner thighs connected. Keep an eye on your pelvis; it should remain square. Use the inner thighs to help stabilize the hip bones.
- Keeping the navel to the spine is essential.

Go to the Can Can on page 137.

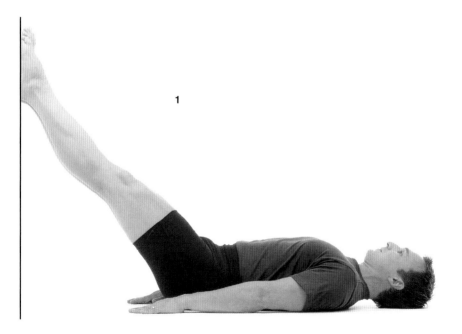

1

Teaser

Transition and Starting Position

From the Torpedo (page 128), roll onto your back with the legs straight out on the mat. The arms are in a low 'V'.

Start Position

- Breathe in to prepare and engage the lower abdominals.
- Breathe out, bend the knees and hinge both legs up over you. Simultaneously, curl the head and shoulders off the mat. The focus is down. The shoulders are down. Keeping a very hollow centre, extend the legs out to about a 45-degree angle from the floor. Keep the back grounded to the mat. Use the mirror to view your profile. **(1)**

Movement

- Breathe in and roll up through the spine, beginning the movement by nodding the head and then breaking from the breastbone. Work through the lower back. The legs stay where you placed them and should not drop towards the mat. Feel the hips, fronts of thighs and abdominals working. Do not let the lower back arch under the weight of the legs.
- The hands aim at the toes. **(2)**
- Breathe out and, starting from the buttocks, roll smoothly back down through the spine, squeezing the inner thighs together. When your shoulder blades reach the mat, stop and roll up again as described above. Once you are strong enough, roll back down to the mat to the start position. (see page 131 **(1)**)
- Do up to 6 smooth rolls.
- To finish, bend the knees in and place the feet on the mat. Roll up through the spine until you are sitting up.

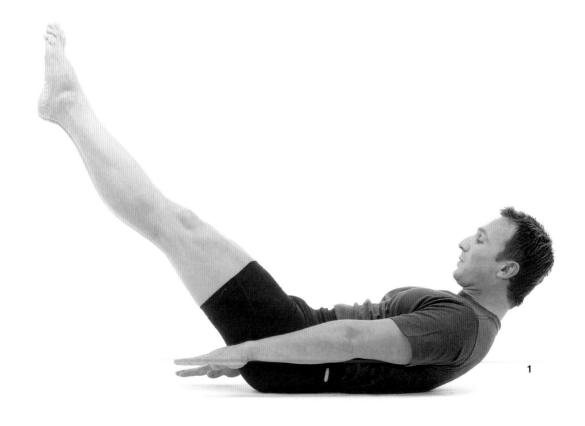

1

Check Points

As for beginners but also:

- Your legs and feet remain fixed in space.
- Press through the lower back.
- Do not allow the weight of the legs to pull the pelvis forward!
- Do not allow the abdominals to bulge.
- Do not hunch the shoulders or close the chest when reaching forward with the hands.
- Your eye focus starts on your centre and then moves to your feet. This will help your balance.
- Keep the pelvis square. This is aided by squeezing the inner thighs.

Go to Hip Twists on page 138.

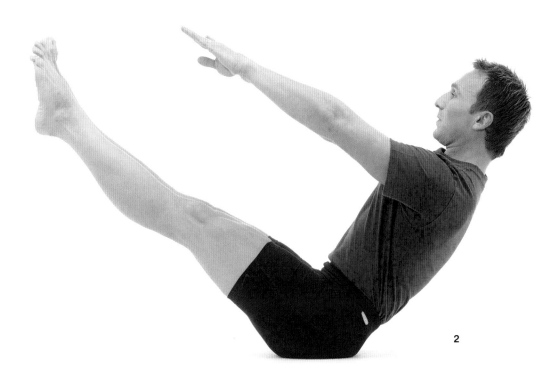

2

Teaser

This is very demanding on the abdominals.
It's easy to cheat using the arms for momentum!

Transition and Starting Position

From the Torpedo (page 129), roll onto your back, making sure you are in the centre of your mat, and bring the arms above the head, resting them on the mat behind you. Use the mirror in profile. **(1)**

Movement

- Breathe out to prepare, hollowing navel to spine.
- Breathe in and lift the arms and the head and roll up through the spine, simultaneously lifting the legs straight up off the mat. **(2 and 3)**
- The arms stay by the ears as you form the 'V'. **(4)**
- This demands a great deal of work in the upper back as you try to straighten it up and a very strong centre. Lower the arms to shoulder height if this is too difficult. **(5)**
- Breathe out and roll back down through the spine, keeping the arms level with your ears. The feet and head should arrive back on the mat at the same time. **(4 to 1)**
- Repeat up to 6 times.

Check Points

As for intermediates but also:

- Try to keep the shoulders away from your ears.
- Do not whip the arms forward and use their momentum to aid the roll-up. They stay close to the head.
- Think of lifting the breastbone up as you form the 'V'.
- Do not allow the back to arch as you lift up into the 'V'. Initiate the movement with the arms and head and then lift the legs.

Go to Hip Twists on page 139. ➡

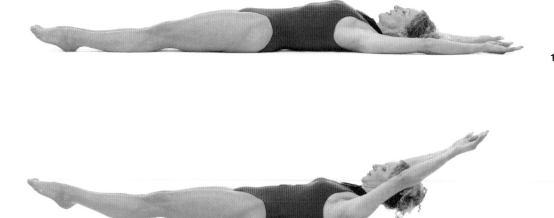

1

2

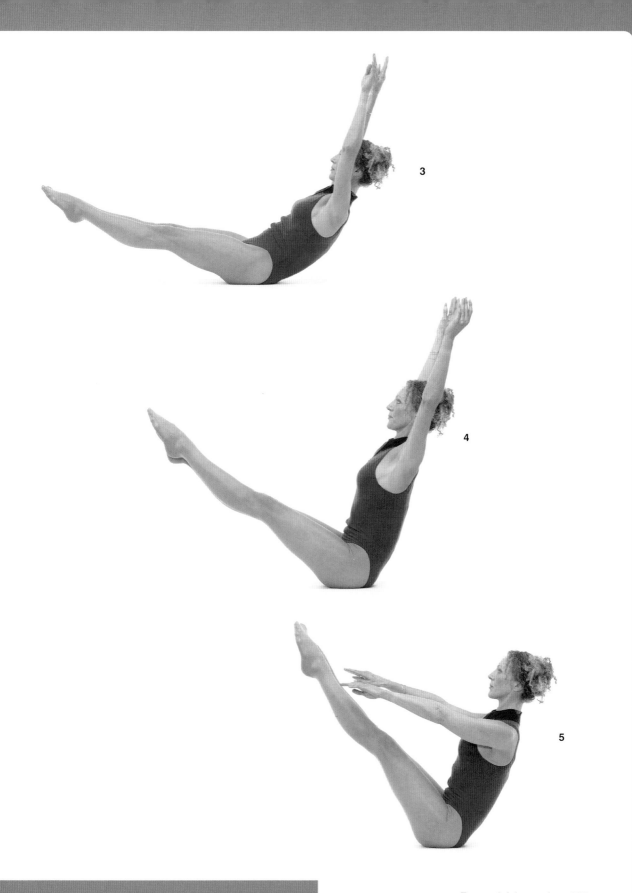

3

4

5

Hip Twists

Aim

To strengthen the hips, the fronts of the thighs and the abdominals.

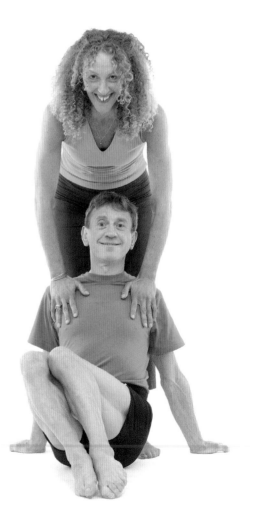

Can Can

This is a preparatory exercise for Hip Twists, where you practise keeping the upper body still as the hips move.

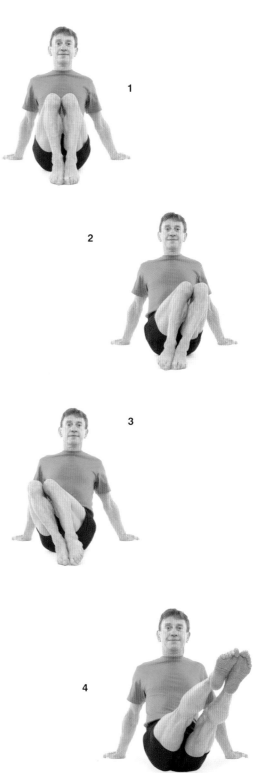

Starting Position

Sit up with the legs bent in front of you and the inner thighs connected. Place the hands behind you, slightly wider apart than the hips with the fingers pointing backwards. Rock back on your tailbone. Lift the heels off the mat and softly point the toes so they are just touching the mat. Open up across the chest, lifting the breastbone towards the ceiling and hollowing your navel to your spine. Your back should be flat. Your focus is straight ahead. Use the mirror straight ahead of you to check for square shoulders. Put it in profile to check your back is flat and not rounded. **(1)**

Movement

- Breathe in and twist the knees to the left keeping them together. The upper back and chest are absolutely still and square to the front. Feel the hands anchored firmly into the mat with equal pressure on both hands. **(2)**
- Breathe out and repeat the knee twist to the right. **(3)**
- Breathe in and twist them back to the left.
- Breathe out and kick the legs out straight, keeping them glued together. Try not to let them drop towards the floor. Keep the abdominals hollowed and *do not let the lower back arch*! Hold for a few seconds as you exhale completely. **(4)** Bend the knees back in.
- Repeat the 3 twists, moving the knees to the right first, and the kick the other way.
- Do up to 6 sets of 3 twists on each side.

Check Points

- The hips will move but the upper back and chest should remain immobile.
- Do not collapse across the chest. Keep the breastbone lifting to the ceiling.
- Keep the palms open and the hands anchored.
- Do not bend the arms. Lean back further if you have to.
- The lower back must not arch! Do not straighten the legs completely if it causes the pelvis to tilt forward.
- Keep the inner thighs connected.

Go to Swimming on page 141. ⟹

Hip Twists

Transition and Starting Position

From the end position of Teaser (page 132), place your arms behind the hips (as for the beginners' starting position) and, keeping a very strong and hollow centre, straighten the legs out as high off the mat as you can. If the back starts to arch keep the legs a little bent to reduce the leverage. **(1)**

Movement

- Breathe in and move both legs to the right a little.
- Breathe out and circle them slightly down towards the mat. Keep a strong centre!
- Continue to breathe out and finish the small controlled circular motion clockwise. The hips will move but the upper back and chest remain still in space. Use the mirror!
- Breathe in and move the legs slightly to the left.
- Breathe out and start to circle the legs anti-clockwise.
- Do up to 6 circles, 3 in each direction.

Check Points

- Only do very small, controlled circles at first. The back must not arch.
- Keep the toes reaching to the ceiling.
- Keep the inner thighs connected.
- Plant the hands on the mat and keep a good contact with it.
- Do not slouch in the shoulders or let the arms bend.
- Breathe!

Go to Swimming on page 142. ➡

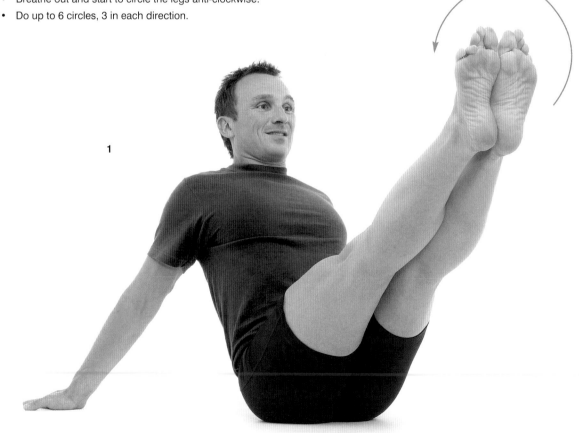

1

Hip Twists

Transition and Starting Position

From the end position of Teaser (see page 134), remain in the 'V' shape, keeping the legs extended out in the air in front of you. Carefully circle the arms up and backwards until the hands reach the mat behind you. They should be slightly wider apart than the hips. **(1)**

Movement

- As for intermediate but make the circles bigger. Only make them as large as you can without losing your centre and your flat back. **(2 to 4)**
- Do up to 6 circles, 3 in each direction.

Check Points

As for the intermediate version. The bigger the circle, the harder it is to keep the back still and the hands planted firmly on the floor.

Go to Swimming on page 143.

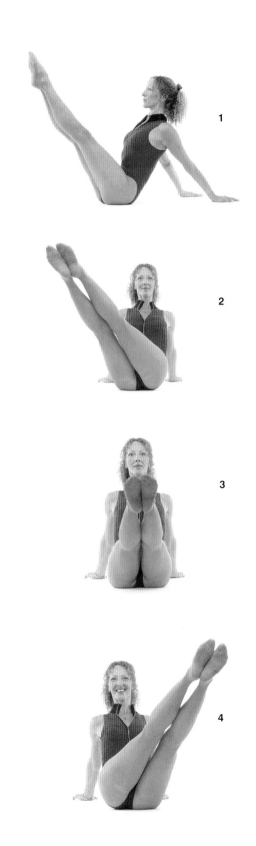

Swimming (Star)

Aim

Having worked hard in the front of the hips, this exercise
helps to stretch out the front of the hips using the opposite
muscle groups at the backs of the thighs and in the
buttocks and emphasizes co-ordination and trunk stability.

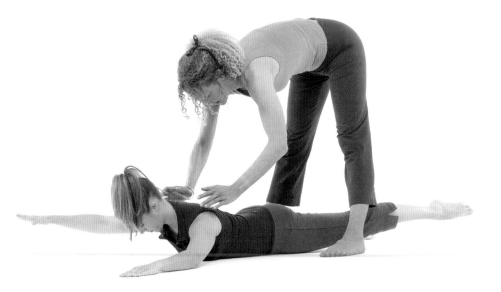

Swimming

This is the preparation for Swimming.

Starting Position

Lie on your front and place a flat cushion under your forehead. Open the legs so they are a little wider apart than the shoulders. Turn the legs out, keeping the knees straight. Stretch the arms above your head on the mat and open them just wider than the shoulders so you are forming a star shape. Draw the shoulders down, away from the ears, and soften the elbows. The palms face down. Make sure you are square on the mat. The mirror can be used straight ahead of you.

Movement

- Breathe in to prepare. Draw the lower abdominals in to the spine.
- Breathe out and lift the right arm just off the mat, keeping the elbow soft and the shoulder down the back. Simultaneously, lift the head and the left leg. Keep the lifts low and the leg straight. The pelvis remains anchored to the mat. Stay long through the lower back. **(1)**
- Breathe in and lower the arm and leg carefully back to the mat and rest the head.
- Do 10 lifts alternating sides.

Check Points

- The pubic bone and both hip bones remain anchored to the mat. Use your buttocks and lower abdominals to help them remain stable.
- Think of opening the front of the shoulder and the hip joints of the limbs you are lifting.
- Keep the back of the neck long and your focus straight down as you lift the head.
- Stretch the leg out of the hip joint.
- The lifts are small. It is not the height which counts, but the stability of the pelvis, torso and shoulders.
- You should feel the work in the back of the thigh, the buttocks and the back.
- Do not allow the abdominals to drop into the mat.

Go to the Seal on page 163. ➡

1

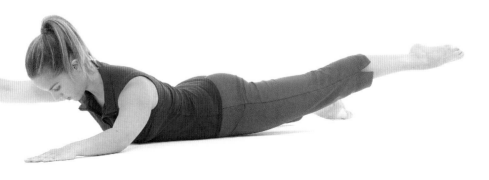

Swimming

Transition and Starting Position

From the last Hip Twist (page 138), bend the legs in, sit up straight and place the arms by your sides. Roll down through the spine, one vertebra at a time. Bring the left arm up by your ear on the floor and roll over towards it. Re-centre yourself on the mat. Bring the legs together with the knees facing the mat and place the arms up above your head. You should be in a straight line, long and slender. Draw the shoulders down the back and scoop in the lower abdominals. Breathe out and lift the right leg, head and left arm just off the mat. Keep the left leg straight and the pubic bone down.

Movement

- Breathe in and, as if swimming, scissor the legs and arms in a small beating motion up and down without touching the mat. **(1)**
- The arms and legs move with smooth control and the torso and pelvis remain still! Count 5 beats.
- Breathe out and count another 5 beats.
- Continue breathing in for 5 and out for 5, until you reach 20 beats. Lower the arms and legs.

Check Points

- Keep this fairly slow.
- Keep the back of the neck long and the back of the skull in line with the spine. Push through the crown of the head if you cannot keep your shoulders down your back, or if you suffer from neck strain.
- The arms remain slightly soft at the elbows, with the palms down.
- The legs will want to bend at the knee. Keep stretching through the backs of the knees. Move from the top of the backs of the thighs and the bottom of the buttocks.
- The body should not move from side to side.

Go to Leg Pull Front on page 145. ➡

1

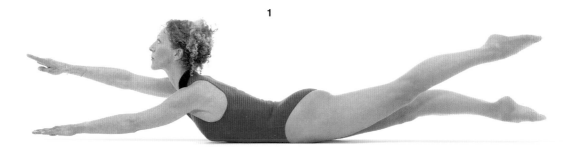

Swimming

Transition and Starting Position

From the last Hip Twist (page 139), lower the legs straight
to the mat with your arms by your sides and roll down
through the spine, as you did in Roll-Ups (page 42). Place
the left arm by your ear on the mat and roll over towards it
bringing the right arm up. Then assume the intermediate
starting position. Breathe out and lift your head, arms and
legs straight off the mat. This time the head is lifted,
looking up. Keep your mouth closed and your shoulders
down away from your ears. Think of being long and thin.
Navel to spine.

Movement

As for intermediate. But this time when you beat the arms
and legs the movement is faster. It will be more difficult to
keep the torso and pelvis still. Use your core stability! **(1)**

Check Points

- As for intermediate, but there is more emphasis on
  keeping the shoulders down and stabilizing the body
  so it does not rock from side to side. The head stays
  up, not aligned with the body as for intermediate.
- Think of moving from the very top of the backs of the
  legs.
- Use the mirror straight ahead of you to check your arm
  and leg movements are equal right and left.

Go to Leg Pull Front on page 146.

1

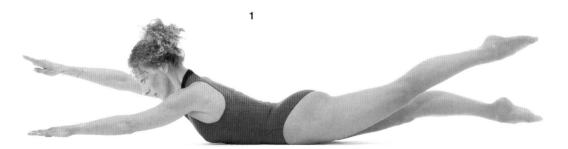

Leg Pull Front

Aim

To strengthen the trunk stabilizers in the stomach, arms, shoulders, buttocks and backs of the legs. Great for runners because it also stretches the calf muscles and the front of the hips.

Leg Pull Front

Transition and Starting Position

From Swimming (page 142), place the hands under the shoulders and brace the abdominals. Breathe out and push up off your hands to come on to your knees. Then sit back on the heels. Stretch for a few deep breaths. Push up into a four-point-kneeling position. The knees are hip-width apart, the hands under the shoulders. The eye focus is straight down. Press up out of the mat firmly into the shoulders without curving the torso. Push the back of the skull towards the ceiling. Have the feet in straight lines. Use the mirror in profile to you. **(1)**

Movement

- Breathe in to prepare and zip up and hollow. Pelvis and spine in neutral.
- Breathe out and slide the right leg directly behind you in line with the hip. Do not allow anything else to move.
- Keep the pelvis steady. Take the weight on the toes of the right foot. **(2)**
- Breathe in and slide the left leg back, taking the weight on both feet. Your body should be like a flat plank. **(3)**
- Breathe out and press both heels back towards the floor, stretching the calves. **(4)**
- Breathe in bringing the heels back over the toes.
- Breathe out and hinge the right leg back in from the hip. Keep the abdominals scooped. Place the right knee back on the mat with the toes pointed. Keep the torso still. Push from the floor into the shoulders to stop them collapsing in towards each other.
- Breathe in and slide the left leg back. You should be back in the four-point-kneeling position. Check your head and shoulder placement. Repeat, leading with the left leg.
- Do the whole exercise 6 times.

Check Points

- Distribute the weight evenly over the hands, knees and toes.
- Do not allow the body to sag when on the toes only. Use your abdominals to support the back. Feel the strength in your thighs and your abdominals.
- Move slowly and with control, keeping the pelvis still in space.

- Stay long from the crown to the tail. Keep the pelvis and spine in neutral.

Go to Leg Pull Back on page 148. ➞

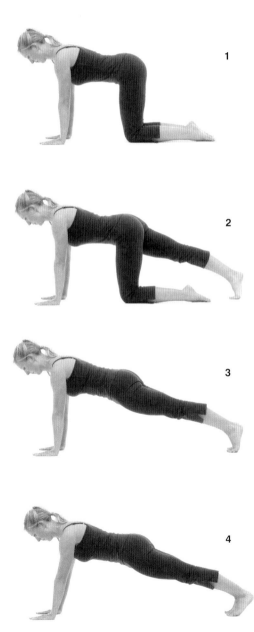

1

2

3

4

Leg Pull Front

A much harder version which needs good strength and body awareness.

Transition and Starting Position

From Swimming (page 143), place the hands under the shoulders, tuck the toes under, straighten the legs and brace the body. Zip up and hollow. Breathe out and push into the hands, lifting the body up off the mat so you finish resting on the hands and the toes. Check your alignment. Look in the mirror to make sure you are not sagging or drooping your head. Look down the body to check the hips are level and the feet are in good alignment. Return the head to centre and push the crown away. **(1)**

Movement

- Breathe in and lift the left leg straight up without moving the pelvis or breaking at the hips. **(2)** Simultaneously, push the right heel down towards the mat, stretching through the Achilles tendon. You may not be able to lift the left leg very far but you must keep it straight. Stretch through the back of the knee, keep a strong leg and the tailbone tucked in. **(3)**
- Breathe out and lower the left leg, continuing to push into the right heel and then return to the starting position. **(4)**
- Breathe in and lift the right leg, pushing into the left heel.
- Do 6 lifts alternating legs.

Check Points

- As for intermediate, the hips must not move.
- Use the back of the leg and the buttock to lift the leg and think of pressing the pelvis forward to the floor to help resist the back pull of the rising leg. Use the mirror to view your profile.
- Do not collapse into the shoulders.
- Do not let the head drop forward.
- Press the crown away from the heels.
- Watch the hips do not hike up to the ribs on the supporting leg side. The Achilles stretch must not affect the hips. Do a couple and look underneath at your hips.

Go to Leg Pull Back on page 150. ➡

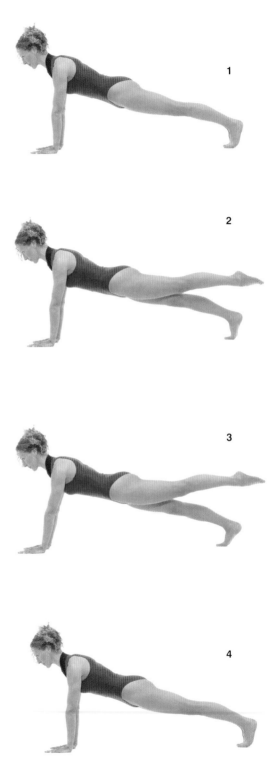

Leg Pull Back

Aim
To work the buttocks, the backs of the legs and the trunk
stabilizers in the back. To strengthen the front of the hips
and the thighs, and the arms and shoulders.

Leg Pull Back

Transition and Starting Position

From the four-point-kneeling position of Leg Pull Front (page 145), simply turn over and sit up with the legs stretched out in front of you. Place the hands on the mat slightly behind the hips with the fingers pointing straight forwards if possible. If this hurts your wrists, leave the fingers pointing backwards. Engage the inner thighs. Imagine a needle is pricking your bottom and lift the hips up so you make a straight line from shoulders to feet. The feet are softly pointed and the knees point straight upwards. Look at your profile in the mirror and check your bottom is not drooping towards the mat. Feel the buttocks and the backs of the legs supporting you and feel that you are open across the chest. **(1)**

Movement

- Breathe in and slowly draw the right leg in towards you, keeping the foot sliding along the mat and bending at the knee. Watch out for correct leg alignment! You are now supported by the left leg only. Keep the hips square and the navel to spine. **(2)**
- Breathe out and slide the right foot back out to join the left foot.
- Breathe in and repeat with the left leg, supporting your weight with the right.
- Breathe out and slide the left leg back.
- Do 6 alternating slides.

1

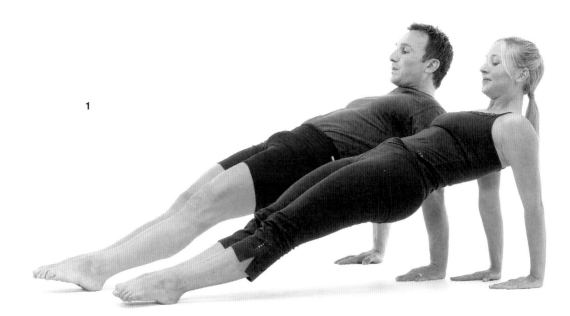

Check Points

- The body must stay in a straight line and the hips remain square.
- Do not sink into the chest and shoulders. Lift up away from the mat.
- Eye focus should be down along the body watching for any unwanted movement of the pelvis.
- Keep the elbows slightly soft so you do not lock them.
- Be careful not to lock the knee joint of the supporting leg. It should be straight and the muscles should be engaged, pulling the kneecap up towards the hips. This will help protect the joint. The backs of the knees should not bend towards the floor.

Go to the Mermaid on page 155.

2

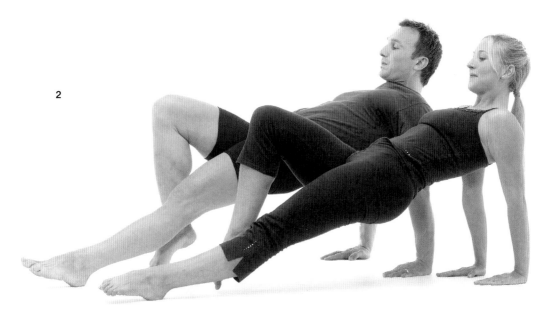

Leg Pull Back

This version makes it much harder to control the pelvis and keep the hips lifted. It is a rhythmical exercise.

Transition and Starting Position

From the last Leg Pull Front (page 146), leave the left hand on the mat and lift the right hand and arm out, away from you, circling it behind you. This will ultimately rotate the chest and the hips so your body faces the ceiling. Place the right hand on the mat under the right shoulder. Throughout these movements, your hips stay lifted and your body is like a plank. The feet will cross, so uncross them as you place the right hand back on the mat. Adjust the fingers so they point straight forwards. Lift the chest and focus down the body. Squeeze the buttocks and the inner thighs. **(1)** Try and make all this a smooth movement! If it is too difficult, do the intermediate transition.

Movement

- Breathe in and kick the right leg straight up *briskly*, keeping stretched through the knee and toes and very still in the body. Do not allow the bottom to drop towards the mat! **(2)** Flex the right foot at the height of the kick.
- Breathe out and *slowly* lower the right leg back down, leading with the heel until it just touches the mat. **(3)**
- Breathe in and kick the left leg up *briskly*, flexing the foot at the top.
- Breathe out and lower *slowly*.
- Either do 6 kicks alternating legs or 3 on one leg and then 3 on the other.

Check Points

- Only kick as high as you can, keeping the bottom lifted and the pelvis and back still.
- Lengthen out of the hip joints.
- Squeeze the buttocks on the supporting side and feel the back of the leg working.
- Keep the knees pointing straight upwards, they should not turn out to the sides.
- Do not collapse across the chest. Keep the arms long.
- Use your breathing to help.

Go to Side Kick Kneeling on page 152. ➡

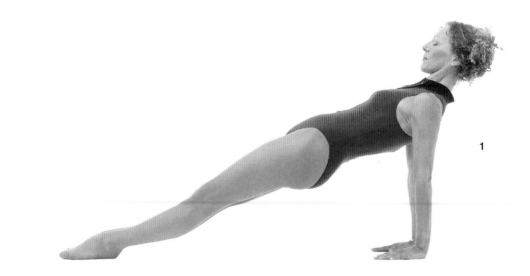

1

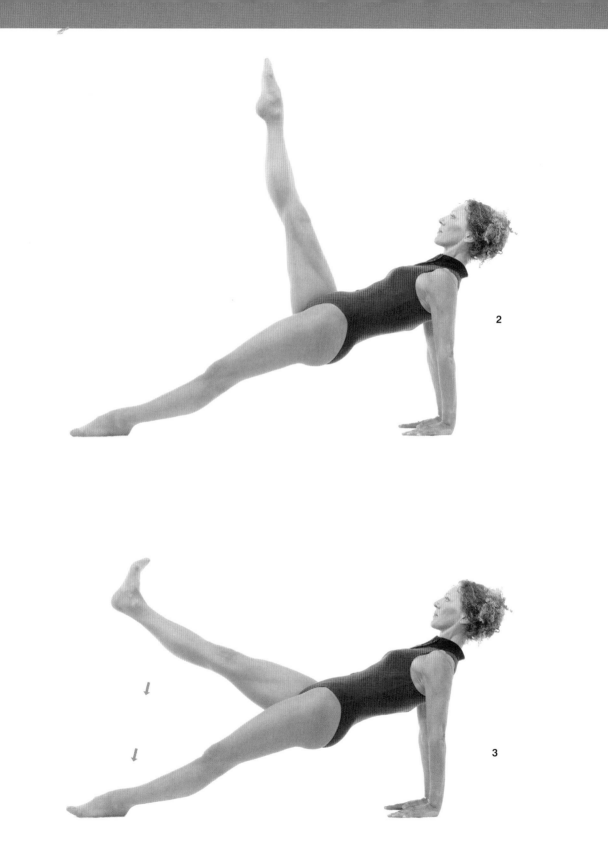

2

3

Side Kick Kneeling

Aim

This exercise is a repeat of Side Kicks (page 121), but with less contact points on the mat and therefore a demand for greater trunk stability. It aims to improve core stability and work the hips. It stretches the front of the hips and the backs of the legs.

Transition and Starting Position

From the last Leg Pull Back (page 150), lower the sit bones on to the mat and bend the knees to the right and roll on to the right hip. Come up to a kneeling position facing sideways on the mat, with the knees under the hips and the arms at your sides. **(1)** Incline to your right and place the right hand on the mat, under the shoulder. Simultaneously extend the left leg out to the side, lifting it directly in line with the hip. Keep long in the waistline. Place the left hand over your right ear and open the elbow. Check your alignment. There should be a straight line through the shoulder to the side of the foot. **(2)**

Movement

- Breathe in and kick the left leg forward exactly as you did in Side Kicks (page 121), flexing the foot at the limit of the kick. **(3)**
- Breathe out and draw the leg backwards, pointing the foot. Do not allow the back or the pelvis to move! **(4)** Do up to 6 kicks on this side.
- To change legs, stretch the left arm up and out in an arc as you bring the left leg in under the body and return the trunk back over the hips. Pause for a split second in the kneeling-up position, **(1)** then incline onto the left hand and extend the right leg up and out in line with the hip.
- Do 6 kicks with each leg.

Check Points

- Keep a very strong centre.
- Look straight ahead of you and lengthen through the crown of the head.
- The hip should be over the knee on the supporting side. **(2)**
- Keep the palm and shin firmly anchored on the mat throughout.
- Do not arch the back. Close the ribcage down.
- Keep the movement smooth and steady.
- Start by doing very few.

Go to the Twist on page 156. ➡

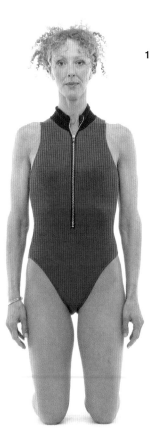

1

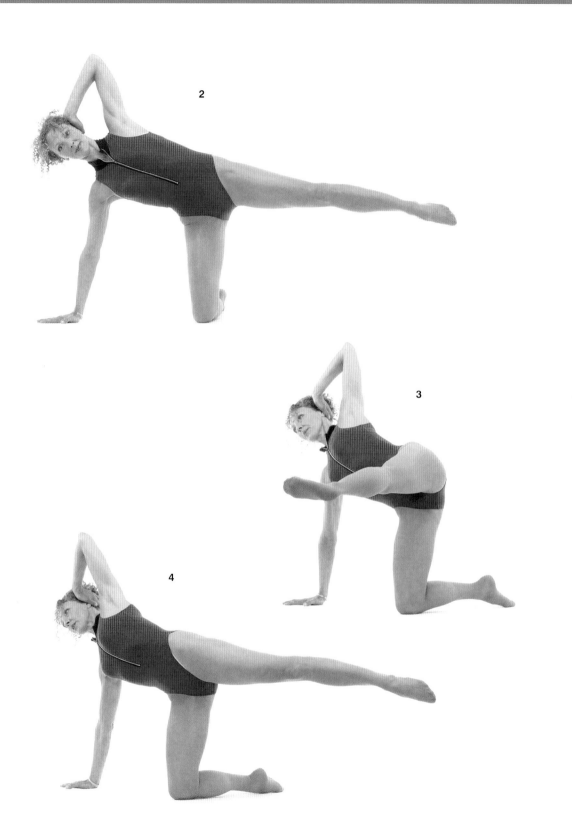

2

3

4

The Twist

Aim

To gain control, grace and balance, to cinch in the
waistline and to stretch the sides

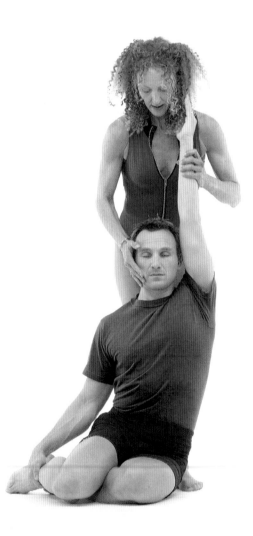

The Mermaid

Transition and Starting Position

From the last Leg Pull Back (page 148), lower the hips to the mat, bend the knees and kneel back onto the heels, facing sideways on the mat with the length of the mat on your left. Drop the left hip on to the mat, trying to keep your legs together, like a mermaid's tail. In order to balance and be comfortable you might have to adjust the legs away a little. There should be no pain in the knees or hips. Hold the feet with your right hand and raise your left arm up beside your ear, lengthening up out of the hips. **(1)**

Movement

- Breathe out and stretch over towards the right. This stretches the ribs and the left hip. Melt down towards the feet. **(2)**
- Breathe in and come back to the centre, circling the left arm up and over to place it on the mat a little way away from your left hip; your body will incline to the left. **(3)**
- Breathe out and lower the elbow to the mat as you lift the right arm up in an arc over your head. Keep a long waistline on both sides.
- Breathe in and, keeping a strong centre, lift the hips straight off the mat. Keep square to the front. Try to make an arc with the body. **(4)**
- Breathe out and lower the hips back to the mat with control.
- Breathe in and, pressing down into the mat with the left arm and circling the right up and out to the right, start returning to centre. Keep long in the spine and up out of the hips.
- Breathe out as you settle back on to the left hip and hold the feet again.
- Breathe in and lift the left arm back up to your ear, ready to start again. **(5)**
- Repeat 3 times. Change sides with the length of the mat to your right and repeat 3 more times.

Check Points

- Keep the head in alignment with the spine.
- On the first stretch, keep the arm on the ear or as close to the head as possible.
- Keep the back supported by the abdominals.
- Do not sink into the shoulder when supported on the forearm. Keep in a straight line.

- Do not flare the ribs or allow the back to arch on the second stretch.

Go to the Seal on page 162.

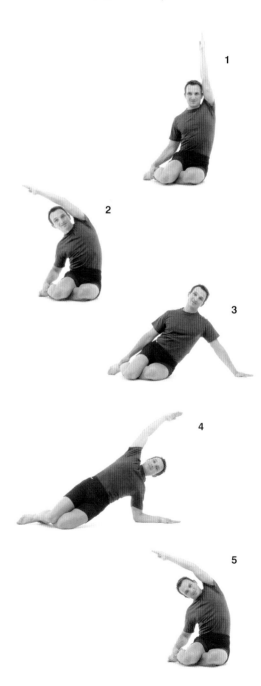

The Twist

Transition and Starting Position

From the last Side Kick Kneeling (page 152), come to the kneeling-up position. Sit on your left hip and place the left hand on the floor a little way from the left hip and in line with it. The fingers should point slightly forward. Slide the left knee forward a little so the left foot is in line with your hips. The left leg is bent and the left foot about 40 centimetres away from your crotch. Move the right foot over the left ankle and plant it firmly on the mat with the toes pointing slightly forwards. Lift the right knee up and open it. Place the right arm out to rest on the right knee. Look straight ahead of you. Your torso and hips should be facing the side. Draw in the lower abdominals ready to move. **(1)**

Movement

- Breathe in and raise the right arm up and over your head in line with the ear as you lift the hips straight up, keeping the pelvis facing forward. The legs will straighten as you push up into a high arc. **(2)** Exhale completely and twist the upper body towards the mat. Reach your right arm under the left and keeping the right arm close to your right ear. Squeeze the inner thighs, keeping the pelvis facing as squarely to the front as possible. **(3)** Lift the pelvis higher towards the ceiling by pulling backwards towards the feet and upwards. Keep the upper body twisting under you and the arm close to the ear. You should feel a deep contraction on the underneath waistline and a stretch over the right side of the trunk. **(4)**
- Breathe out and unwind slowly lowering the hips back to the mat to the starting position.
- Repeat 3 times, then turn to face the other side and repeat the movement 3 times.

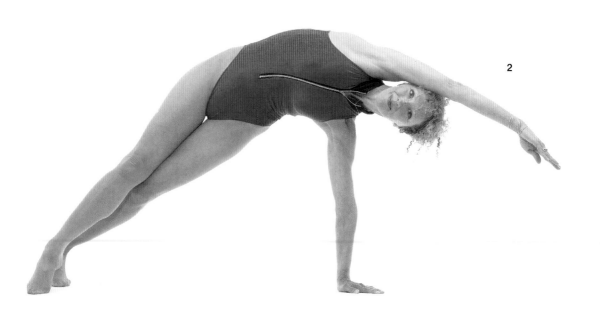

1

2

Check Points

- The buttocks, inner thighs and abdominals all need to work to hold the balance.
- You should feel a stretch along the upper side of the body and a deep contraction on the underside.
- Keep the pelvis square and facing the front.
- Do not sink into the supporting shoulder.

- Do not allow the upper arm to swing out behind the body. Keep it in line and near the ear during the stretch under.
- As you lower back to the mat, keep the shoulders down the back and do not plonk on to it.
- Breathe!

Go to Boomerang on page 158.

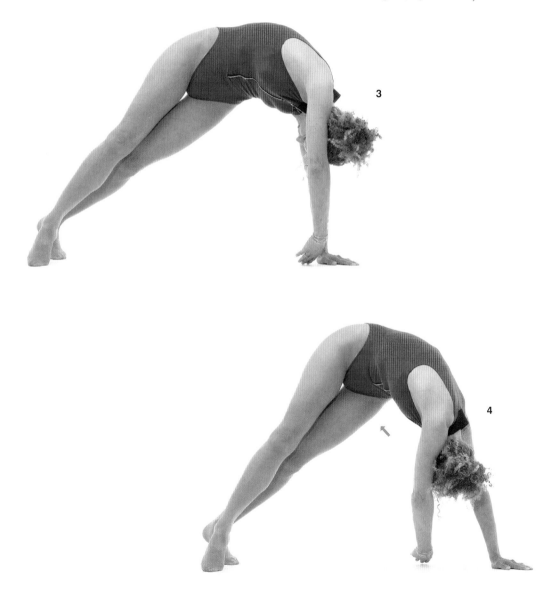

3

4

Boomerang

Aim

To incorporate all the principals of the technique into a smooth flowing motion. This exercise is a choreographed sequence of movements.

Transition and Starting Position

From the last Twist (page 156), sit back squarely on the sit bones and stretch the legs out in front of you. Cross the right leg over the left and squeeze the thighs together. Both legs are straight and turned out, so the knees face outwards. Place the hands next to your hips with the fingers pointing forward. Scoop out the abdominals. Sit right up out of the hips and contract the buttocks. Keep a straight back. **(1)**

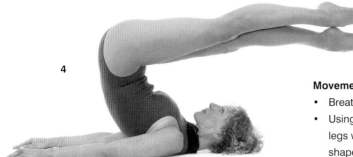

4

Movement

- Breathe out and drop the eye focus down.
- Using the hands to help, rock backwards and lift the legs without breaking the angle at the hips. Keep the shape! Use your stomach! Roll through the spine until you are resting on the shoulders and the legs are right over the body. **(2 to 4)**
- Breathe in and open and close the legs briskly, switching the left leg over the right, like scissors. **(5)** Lift the arms off the mat so you are balancing on the shoulders. **(6)**
- Breathe out and, keeping the chin in and the focus on your centre, roll back up to form a 'V'. Stretch the toes to the ceiling and lift the chest. The arms reach forward to the toes. Hold the position. Look straight ahead. **(7)**

5

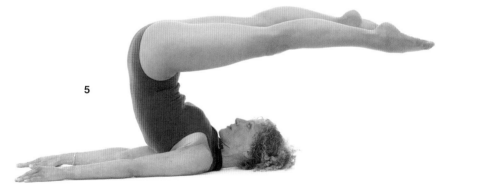

6

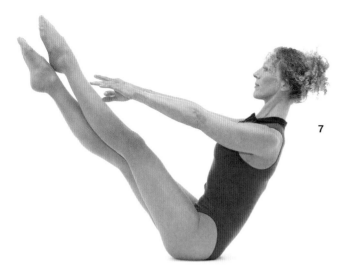

7

- Breathe in and circle the arms out and round behind
  your back. The palms face backwards. Keep a firm
  centre and the chest open. **(8 to 9)**
- If you can, clasp the hands behind your back with
  the palms facing your back, and press them up to
  the ceiling.
- Breathe out and hold the shape. Slowly lower the legs
  to the mat bringing the body forward with the legs, so
  the angle at the hips remains constant. Keep the arms
  reaching up and over the back of your head. **(10 to 11)**
  Fold the body over the legs as you release the hands
  and circle the arms further up towards the ceiling and
  then out and round until they reach out over the legs.
  Try to get your nose on your knees while keeping the
  abdominals drawn in! **(12)**

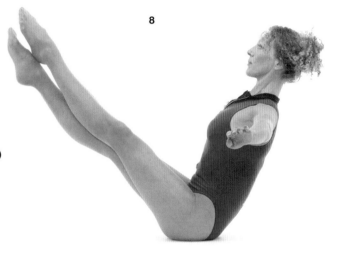

8

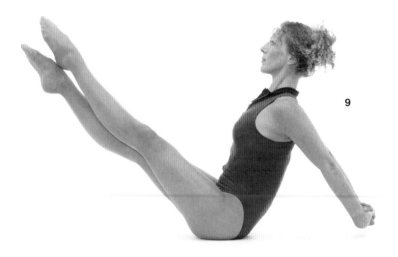

9

- Breathe in and roll up through the spine to the starting position. **(13)** The arms settle back alongside the hips and the shoulders drop back down the spine. Place the hands firmly on the mat. Your left leg is now on top of the right.
- Repeat the whole sequence, switching the legs while balancing on the shoulders.
- Do up to 6 repetitions.

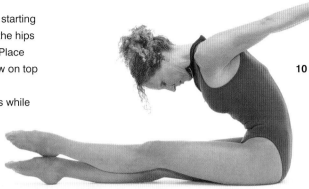

10

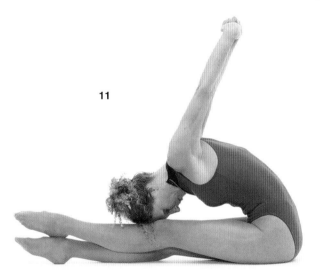

11

Check Points

- Do not lose your centre. Keep the abdominals hollowed throughout.
- Switch the legs briskly and reconnect the inner thighs.
- As you roll up to the 'V', keep the chin tucked in and the focus down until you straighten the spine and open the chest. Only then should your focus shift out to the feet.
- If you cannot clasp the hands, just get them as close together as you can.
- When circling the arms, really work to keep the circle big and smooth and the shoulders stabilized.
- Keep the inner thighs squeezing together. Keep the pelvis square.

Go to the Seal on page 163. ⟹

12

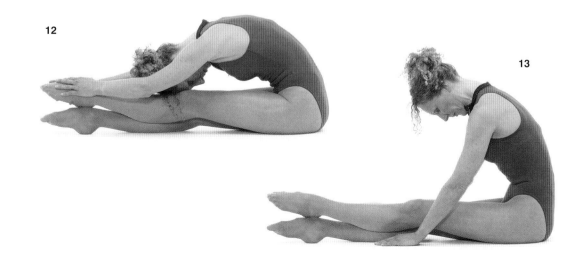

13

The Seal

Aim

This rolling exercise opens the hips, massages the spine and uses the core for balance and control.

Starting Position (beginners)

Sit up on the mat with the knees bent. Rock back on the tailbone, hollowing the lower abdominals, rounding the back and opening the knees. Weave your arms through the inside of the legs and wrap your hands round the tops of the feet. Press the soles of the feet together. Note how you have to open up the hips. Find a place of steady balance and focus down on your pelvis. In spite of the position of the arms, try to open the elbows to create an open chest. Draw the shoulders down the back. **(1)**

Transition and Starting Position (intermediate)

From the last Twist (page 155), turn back to face the front of the mat, keeping the legs bent. Proceed as described in the beginners' version.

Transition and Starting Position (advanced)

From the last Boomerang (page 158), simply stay sitting up, bend the knees in and proceed as for beginners to assume the starting position with the soles of the feet pressed together.

Movement (beginners)

- Breathe in and roll back through the spine. This is done by pulling the sit bones under, not by throwing the head back. Keep your feet the same distance from your crotch throughout. Use those abdominals! Roll no further than the shoulders, keeping the head and neck off the mat. **(2)**
- Breathe out and roll back up continuing to press the soles of the feet together and keeping exactly the same shape.
- Do 6 smooth, controlled rolls.

Check Points (beginners)

- The main ways of cheating are to throw the head back to move and to let the legs slightly lengthen, pulling the feet away from the crotch. Neither must happen.
- Keep the abdominals pressing into the spine.
- Keep the focus down throughout.
- Control the roll back so you balance on your shoulders.
- Do not hunch the shoulders at any time.
- When rolled up do not move the chest or the pelvis. Keep in the curled position.

The Seal

Movement (intermediate and advanced)

- As for beginners, except that when you have found the place of balance on the shoulders, clap the soles of the feet together 3 times moving from the hips, and repeat the claps once you have rolled forward and are balanced on the tailbone. This ensures you have found your centre and demands more control.
- Breathe in, roll back and clap the feet 3 times.
- Breathe out, roll forward and then clap the feet 3 times.
- Do 6 complete rolls and finish balanced on the tailbone.

Check Points (intermediate and advanced)

Same as for beginners but also:

- Hold your centre when clapping, the movement of the legs will affect your balance.
- Keep pressing the soles of the feet together while rolling, it opens the hips up and helps maintain the shape.
- The entire foot claps, not just the balls of the feet.
- Watch out for body symmetry.

Go to Rocking on page 165.
Go to Rocking on page 166.

1

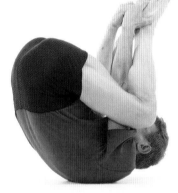

2

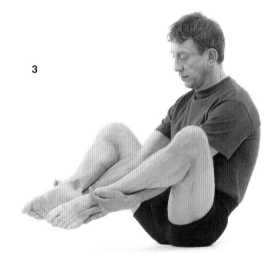

3

Congratulations
to those of you doing the essential exercises and beginners' levels. This is the final exercise in your programme.

Rocking

Aim

To stretch the whole of the front of the body – ankles to thighs, hips, abdominals and neck!

Rocking

Transition and Starting Position

From the last roll forward of the Seal (page 163), carefully lower the feet to the mat. Stretch the legs out a little, bringing the knees together. Place the arms by your sides. Roll down onto the mat through the spine one vertebra at a time. Place your right arm up by your ear and roll over towards it onto your front. Square yourself up on the mat. Lie in a straight line with the left cheek down on the mat. Then lift the head, bend the right leg and reach behind you to grasp the right foot with the right hand. Bend the left leg and grasp the left foot with the left hand. Make sure your lower abdominals are pulled in to the spine! Bring the knees together and anchor the pubic bone to the mat. **(1)**

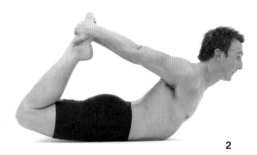

Movement

- Breathe in and, really drawing the abdominals in, pull the feet away from your back so the chest lifts and opens and the back arcs. The knees should lift up off the mat and they will open a little. Feel the stretch across the chest, the front of the hips and the thighs. The buttocks, the backs of the legs and the back muscles are all working. Use the mirror in front of you. **(2)**
- Breathe out and lower the knees and chest back down releasing the pull. Lower the head on to the other cheek. Press the pubic bone to the mat and ease the feet into the buttocks. Feel the stretch down the front of the thighs.
- Do 6 stretches.

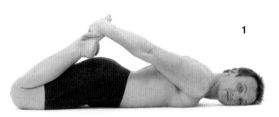

Check Points

- **It is imperative not to let the navel push down into the mat as you arc up.**
- Let the pull of the legs open the front of the shoulders without allowing the shoulder to hunch.
- Get a good grip with the hands.
- Check in the mirror to see if the shoulders, legs and feet are symmetrical.
- Do not worry if you cannot pull up very high off the mat. It will come as you practise.

Go to the last exercise, the Push-Up on page 172 ➡

Rocking

Transition and Starting Position.

As for the intermediate version, but you roll down through the spine with straight legs together, and flexed feet. Roll over onto your front and assume the starting position described in the intermediate version.

Movement

- Breathe in and press the feet into your hands to lift the legs and back into the arc. Imagine the rockers on a rocking chair. **(1)**
- Breathe out and kick back into the hands to produce the motion to start rocking backwards. Lift the chin to the ceiling. You are strung out like a bow. **(2 and 3)**
- Breathe in and rock forward on to the breastbone, keeping the chin lifted. **(4)** Breathe out and push into the hands again to lift back up. **(3)**
- Once you have the momentum going, hold the pull of the legs to keep the shape you have made. Do not collapse on the rock forward.
- Do up to 6 rocks.

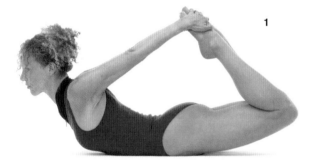

1

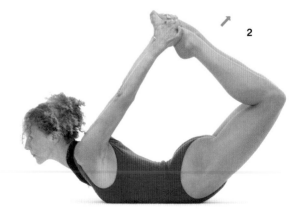

2

Check Points

- Do not rock the head to and fro to move. Use the legs and the back.
- Keep the abdominals pulled into the spine. Keep the tension pulled out between the arms and the legs as you rock forward.
- Do not allow the knees to open right out. Try and keep them in line with the hips. Use the mirror.
- Do not shorten in the back of the neck.
- Keep the shoulders down.
- Do not push the abdominals into the mat, keep navel to spine.
- Once you can achieve a steady rock and no longer need the mirror, you can have your chin lifted throughout the exercise taking the whole body into extension.

Go to Control and Balance on page 168. ➡

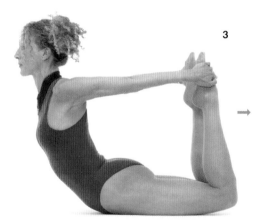

3

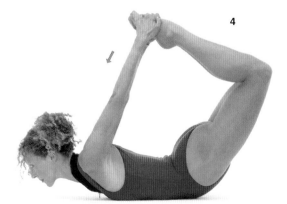

4

Control and Balance

Aim

This exercise trains the centre to maintain balance and support the spine. It is very hard to have control without cheating by using the head and neck to balance.

Transition and Starting Position

From the last Rocking (page 166), release the legs and hands and lie straight on the mat on your front. Bring the right arm up and roll over onto your back, centring yourself in the middle of the mat. Place both arms above your head on the mat and bring the legs in towards your chest keeping them bent and squeezed together. Straighten the legs straight up to the ceiling and then, breathing out, roll the spine off the mat as you did during Roll Over (page 47). Try to keep the toes just off the mat behind your head. Grasp the right ankle in both hands. **(1)**

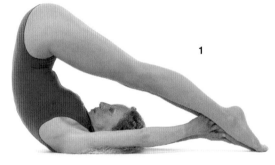

1

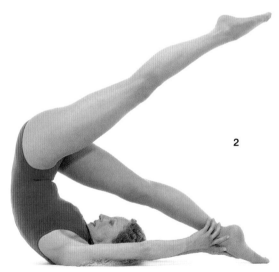

2

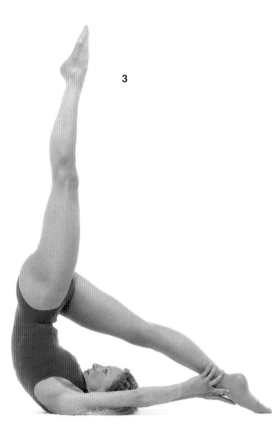

3

Movement

- Breathe in and slowly raise the left leg, reaching the toes to the ceiling. Keep the pelvis square. Try to bring the foot directly over the left hip. **(2 and 3)**
- Breathe out, release your right foot and raise your right leg up, simultaneously lowering the left leg down and grasping the left ankle. **(4 to 6)** Stretch the right leg up, lifting out of the hips, toes trying to touch the ceiling. Keep the legs in alignment with the hip sockets or sit bones. **(7)** The pelvis stays square and still. Watch it. Use your centre to balance. Do it slowly!
- Breathe in and switch legs again.
- Do 6 changes.

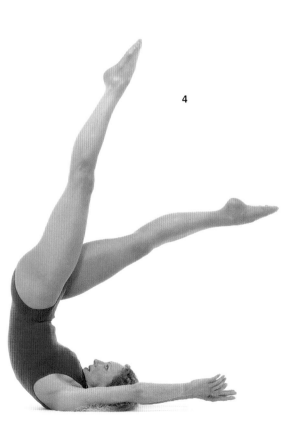

4

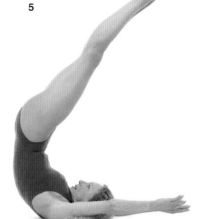

5

- To finish, bring both legs back down so the toes are on or near the mat behind your head and roll the spine back down on to the mat, anchoring through the back of the skull and across the chest. When the pelvis reaches the mat, bend the knees in towards the chest and hinge them back down to the floor. Roll up through the spine to sitting. Stand up and place yourself at the end of the mat, facing it with the feet hip-width apart.

Check Points

- Keep navel to spine and a strong flat centre.
- The knees face straight towards you.
- Lower the legs towards the ear and not across your face or out to the sides. Watch both legs.
- Try not to hunch the shoulders. Keep the collarbone away from the ear lobe.
- Think of pulling the leg up towards the ceiling using the back of the leg and the buttocks.
- Breathe!

Go to the last exercise, the Push-Up on page 176. ➡

6

7

The Push-Up

The grand finale which leaves you standing up,
ready to go forth and conquer!

The Push-Up

Transition and Starting Position

From the last stretch of Rocking (page 165), lie straight out on your front and place your hands under your shoulders. Open the knees to hip-width apart. Brace the abdominals, scooping up below the navel, and push up so the body is like a straight plank from knees to shoulders. Do not let the shoulder blades pinch together or rise up near your ears. As you push off the floor, keep the back of the skull in line with the back and not dropping forward to the floor. **(1)** Breathe in and lift the tailbone up and backwards, as if it is being pulled by a cord from the navel. **(2)** Push back with the arms. Breathe out and push the sit bones back onto your heels leaving the arms stretched out on the mat. Push the chest gently to the floor. **(3)** Keep the neck long and chin down. Breathe in and slide the arms in towards you a little. Breathe out and, starting from the sit bones, tuck the pelvis under and roll up through the spine until you are kneeling up. **(4 to 6)**

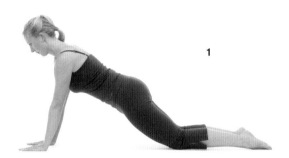

1

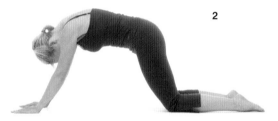

2

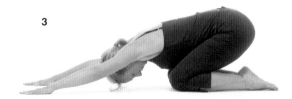

3

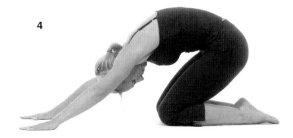

4

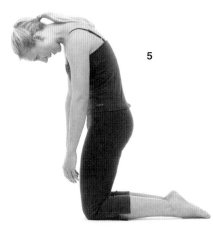

5

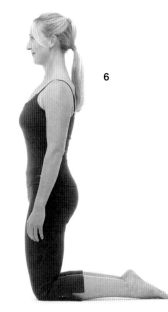

6

Movement

- Breathe in and slowly roll the body down. Start by nodding your head and then break at the breastbone, keeping the pelvis still. **(7)**
- Breathe out when your hands reach the mat **(8)** and walk out on them to form the plank again. **(9)**
- Breathe in and bend the elbows, keeping them close to the body and lowering the rigid torso towards the mat. Keep the shoulders still and the head pushing back to the ceiling. Look straight down. **(10)**
- Breathe out and straighten the arms, lifting the body back.
- Do 3 push-ups breathing in to lower and out to push up.
- Breathe in, tuck the chin and lift the pelvis upwards and backwards. **(11)** Keep the hands planted on the mat and the chest close to it. Stretch the upper back and under the arms. Press the sit bones back towards the heels. **(12)**
- Breathe out, hollow the lower abdominals and drop the tailbone down. Roll up through the spine allowing the arms to slide back along the mat until you are kneeling back up. **(4, 5 and 6)**
- Do a set of 3 push-ups, 4 to 5 times.
- To finish, on the last roll-up to kneeling, rock back on to the feet putting the hands on the floor to help. Scoop out the abdominals and straighten the legs. Breathe out and roll up through the spine until you are standing tall and straight.

Check Points

- You must not sag in the abdominals. Brace them to stay like the plank.
- Watch your head and shoulder alignment. Use the mirror in profile.
- Only bend the arms a little if your shoulders move. Try not to form a cleavage between the shoulder blades! Increase the depth of the push-up as you strengthen.
- Think of tucking the tail under a little when you are in the plank position.
- Do not push your nose to the mat. The head remains still and in line with the spine.

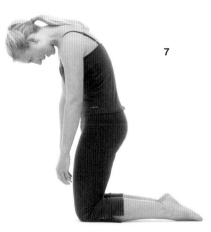

7

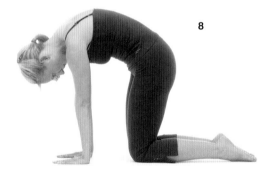

8

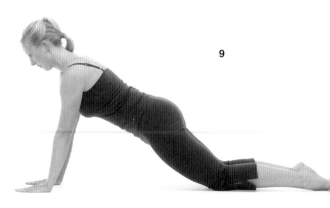

9

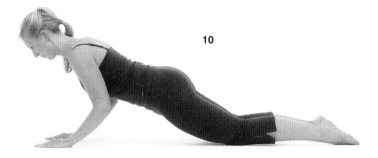

10

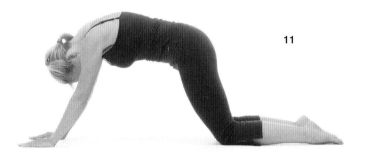

11

12

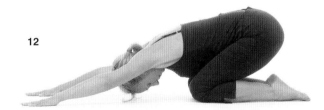

Congratulations!
You have finished
the intermediate mat
programme.

The Push-Up

Transition and Starting Position

From Control and Balance (page 168), you should be
standing tall with the mat in front of you. The feet should
be on the mat. **(1)**

Movement

- Breathe in and roll down through the spine keeping
  your head close to the body and legs as you go.
  Tuck your head in towards your shins! **(2 and 3)**
- Breathe out when the hands reach the mat and walk
  them out keeping the heels pushed into the floor and
  the sit bones lifted. **(4)** Feel the stretch in the backs of
  the legs and the upper back. Keep your abdominals
  pulled in. **(5)**
- When the heels have to lift, bring the shoulders forward
  over the hands to form a long, flat plank, with only the
  hands and toes to support you. **(6)**

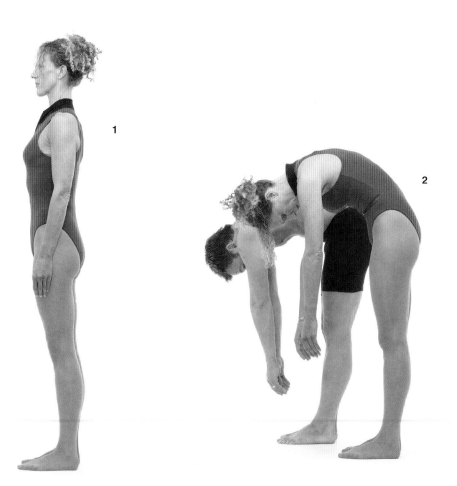

1

2

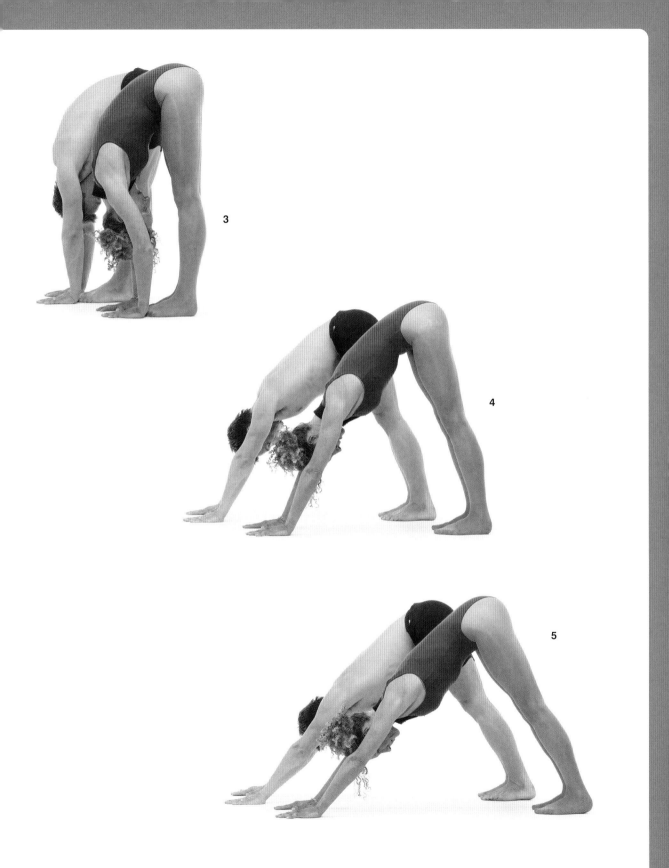

3

4

5

- Breathe in and bend the elbows.
- Keep the arms brushing the body as you lower and the elbows pointing straight back. This is a triceps push-up. **(7)**
- Breathe out and push up, straightening the arms.
- Do 3 push-ups.
- Breathe in, tuck the chin in and start walking the hands back towards your feet. Simultaneously, lift from the navel, pushing the sit bones back up to the ceiling and pressing the heels back towards the floor. **(8)** Bring your head as close to your shins as possible. **(3)**
- Breathe out and walk the hands back up the legs and body. Roll up through the spine to the standing starting position. **(3, 2 and1)**
- Do a set of 3 push-ups up to 5 times.

Check Points

- Keep your head close to your body as you roll down.
- Watch your foot alignment.
- Keep a firm, flat centre, supporting the spine.
- Press the crown of your head away from the heels.
- This is a triceps push-up and very hard to perform correctly. The shoulders must not move. Keep them down the back and think of wrapping the shoulder blades round and under the armpits. Put the weight through both hands, not just your strong arm.
- Do not waddle on the walk out and back on the hands. Follow a straight line.
- Really scoop out the abdominals. You must not sag in the middle. Use the mirror in profile.

Congratulations!
You have finished the full advanced mat programme. Go and take a shower! You should be feeling great but sweating!

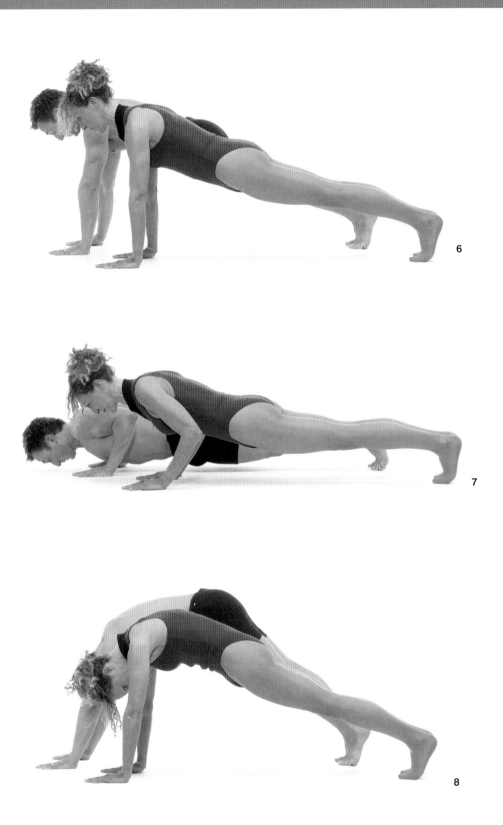

6

7

8

Further Information

For details of your nearest Body Control Pilates teacher, plus a wide range of Pilates equipment, books, videos and accessories, send a stamped addressed envelope to:

The Body Control Pilates Association
PO Box 29061
London WC2H 9TB
England
+44 (0) 20 7379 3734

Or visit the Body Control Pilates website at
www.bodycontrol.co.uk

To contact Miranda Bass
telephone: 01883 742257
www.basspilates.com

Exercise clothing by Asquith Clothing
PO Box 31585
London W11 1ZR
www.asquith.ltd.uk

Watch out for new titles!

Other Body Control Pilates books

BODY CONTROL THE PILATES WAY
0 330 36945 8 / £7.99

THE MIND–BODY WORKOUT
0 330 36946 6 / £12.99

PILATES THE WAY FORWARD
0 330 37081 2 / £12.99

THE OFFICIAL BODY CONTROL PILATES MANUAL
0 330 39327 8 / £12.99

PILATES GYM
0 330 48309 9 / £12.99

THE BODY CONTROL PILATES BACK BOOK
0 330 48311 0 / £9.99

THE BODY CONTROL PILATES
POCKET TRAVELLER
0 330 49106 7 / £4.99

INTELLIGENT EXERCISE WITH PILATES & YOGA
0 333 98952 X / £16.99

THE PERFECT BODY THE PILATES WAY
0 330 48953 4 / £12.99

PILATES PLUS DIET
0 330 48954 2 / £10.99

These are available from all good bookshops, or can be ordered direct from:
Book Services By Post
PO Box 29
Douglas
Isle of Man IM99 IBQ

Credit card hotline +44 (0) 1624 675 137
Postage and packing free in the UK

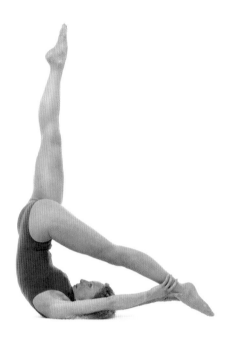

I hope you will really enjoy this unique form of exercise and will be rewarded by good health, a limber body and a stimulated and clear mind, so you are equipped with the strength and endurance we all need to cope with whatever life throws at us.

Remember, it takes time to accomplish the full programme and even the beginners' introductory exercises. Be patient, persevere and reap the benefits of your hard work and commitment.

I wish you all the very best in your endeavours to improve yourselves in body, mind and spirit.